# THE SOMATIC TOOLBOX

Guidebook, Exercises & Deep-Dive Workbook Activities with a 28-Day Program to Increase Self-Awareness, Heal Trauma, Release Pent-up Emotions & Stress in Just 15 Minutes a Day

## ASHLEY WELLSPRING

### IN COLLABORATION WITH SAMANTHA JONES

**BOOK SQUARE PUBLISHING**

**First Printing Edition, 2024**
Printed in the United States of America
Available from Amazon.com and other retail outlets

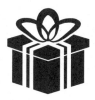

# Your Bonus Material is Here

## Your Somatic Therapy Companions:
## Essential Tools to Transform Your Journey

Right now, as you consider somatic therapy, you should know there's more to it than meets the eye. Sometimes, crucial parts are overlooked, but these are the ones that could really make a big difference for you.

It's about truly understanding yourself and learning to listening to your body and communicate with your emotions. This is what can turn things around.

Our bonuses are designed specifically for that. They're like a bridge between practicing somatic therapy and getting all the benefits from it—making sure you're fully involved in the healing process. Each bonus offers personalized support and tools to help you navigate and transform your emotions, no matter where you are in your journey.

### [BONUS #1] Ecstatic Dance to Release Tension and Emotions Stored in the Body

This audio track is an essential component of a meditative exercise in the workbook, designed specifically to release accumulated emotions and manage stress, promoting a sense of peace and well-being.

### [BONUS #2] Hypnotherapy for Letting Go of the Emotional Pain

Led by Suzanne Robichaud, this hypnotherapy session aims to help you release emotional pain from past experiences and relationships, thereby creating space for increased peace and love.

### [BONUS #3] Guided Meditation for Keeping Yourself Safe During a Dissociative Episode

This meditation is designed to help individuals ground themselves during dissociative episodes. The goal is to foster a sense of safety and facilitate a smooth reintegration with the physical body.

### [BONUS #4] eBook "Body Speaks: How to Understand and Harness Your Emotional Signatures"

You will learn to recognize and interpret your emotional signals, understand what your feelings are communicating, and use these insight to enhance self-awareness and personal growth.

*** Bonus 1, 2, and 3 are designed to enhance the benefits of the 28-day program.

We recommend using them alongside the program to maximize your progress and understanding.

# About This Book

This book is born out of my personal experiences and extensive research in the field of somatic therapy. I wanted to create a practical guide that goes beyond theoretical knowledge - a book that offers actual exercises and a workbook for anyone to start their journey into self-healing at home. While the guidance of a qualified somatic therapist is invaluable, I also understand that the first steps often need to be taken independently. This guide is for those initial steps. It is designed to be a comprehensive but accessible resource: it starts with foundational knowledge, gradually moves into self-awareness and assessment, delves deeper into practical exercises, and finally provides resources for continued learning. It is a safe place to record your experiences, track your progress, and reflect on your learning.

Whether you're dealing with stress, emotional upheaval, physical tension, or just seeking a deeper connection with your inner self, this book offers tools that can be integrated into everyday life. Whether you are a busy professional, a parent balancing numerous responsibilities, someone dealing with the aftermath of emotional or physical trauma, or simply someone who wishes to explore the depths of their being, this guide is for you.

The workbook is structured to facilitate a sequential journey of exploration and discovery. I encourage you to try each exercise, observe how your body and mind respond, and then identify the practices that resonate most with you. This personalized approach ensures that the journey you undertake is uniquely yours, tailored to your own experiences and needs.

1. **Start Sequentially:** Begin with the first exercise and move through them in order. This will give you a comprehensive understanding of the various techniques and their potential impact.

2. **Journal Your Experience:** After each exercise, take a moment to jot down your experiences, thoughts, and feelings. This reflective practice is crucial for deepening your understanding of your body-mind connection.

3. **Identify What Resonates:** As you progress, you'll find certain exercises that resonate more deeply with you. These are the practices that you can integrate more fully into your daily routine.

4. **Repeat and Deepen:** Somatic therapy is a practice. The more you engage with these exercises, the more profound and lasting the benefits will be.

In essence, this book is meant to become the bridge between the world of somatic therapy and your personal journey. Through it, you're not merely reading about healing; you're taking an active role in your own healing process. The power to foster change is in your hands, and as you engage with each exercise, you are stepping closer to the harmony and balance you seek. Embrace it as your stepping stone to a more connected life where your are your own masterful choreographer.

# INTRODUCTION

Imagine for a moment that our bodies and minds are engaged in a complex, beautiful dance. It's not just any dance. In this dance, every step, turn, and jump connects deeply, blending our physical feelings and emotions. Somatic therapy is all about diving deep into this dance. It's about discovering how our bodies and minds talk to each other in a language that's been around longer than any words.

Now, I encourage you to truly grasp this new language, familiarize yourself with the fundamental principles of somatic therapy, and embrace its practices. It is through this deep engagement that you will experience the transformative power of the therapy and the profound changes it can bring into your life.

Before we start, let me share a bit of my own story.

Like so many others, I was deeply entangled in the relentless demands that life so often presents. My days were a balancing act of professional responsibilities and personal commitments. In the corporate world, I was known for my efficiency and reliability, but beneath that composed exterior, stress and anxiety had become my constant, unwelcomed companions.

The mornings began with a heavy sense of dread, a feeling that persisted throughout the day. I remember sitting in endless meetings, my mind fogged with fatigue, struggling to maintain focus. At home, the situation wasn't much better. The simple joys of family life were overshadowed by a persistent sense of overwhelm. I felt like I was always running, yet never really getting anywhere. Every task, whether at work or home, felt like a mountain to climb. I was teetering on the edge of burnout, a state I had read about but never truly understood until I found myself staring it in the face.

The pivotal moment in my life came rather unexpectedly. It wasn't a dramatic breakdown or a health scare, as one might expect. It was a quiet realization during a rare moment of stillness on a particularly challenging day. I noticed that the stress I was experiencing wasn't just a mental or emotional state; it had become a physical sensation, manifesting as a constant tension in my shoulders, a knot in my stomach, a relentless headache. It dawned on me that the weight I was carrying wasn't just mental or emotional; it had seeped deep into my physical being. I had become a living example of the mind-body connection, a concept I had only superficially understood until then.

In this state of heightened awareness, I recognized that I was living, but not thriving. I was surviving, but not flourishing. This realization was both frightening and enlightening. It led me down a path I had never anticipated – the path of somatic therapy.

Turning to somatic therapy wasn't an easy decision. It came from a place of desperation, a longing for change and healing. I began exploring different modalities, I attended workshops, read extensively, and sought the guidance of experts in the field. The more I learned, the more I realized how disconnected I had become from my own body.

Somatic therapy opened my eyes to a world where the body speaks a language of its own, often ignored or misunderstood. As I began to truly listen and tune in to my body, I uncovered layers of wisdom that had been buried under years of neglect and disconnection. The journey was revelatory in many ways. Learning to recognize the subtle cues of tension and release was like learning a new language. I noticed how certain situations or thoughts would trigger a tightening in my chest or a clenching of my jaw. Conversely, moments of joy and relaxation manifested as a sense of lightness, an easy breath, and a feeling of openness in my body. These were not just fleeting physical sensations; they were direct communications from my body, guiding me towards a deeper understanding of my emotional and psychological state. Employing techniques like mindful movement, breathwork, and guided imagery, I began to actively engage with these bodily sensations. Mindful movement, in particular, became a daily ritual. It was a way for me to connect with my body, to express and release emotions through physical activity. Breathwork helped me regulate my responses to stress, bringing a sense of calm and focus that was previously elusive. Guided imagery served as a bridge, connecting my conscious and subconscious mind, allowing me to explore and release deep-seated emotions and traumas.

The practical benefits of this journey were profound and multifaceted. Physically, the chronic tension that I had carried for years began to unravel. My posture improved, and with it, the recurrent backaches and muscle stiffness reduced significantly. The quality of my sleep improved, no longer disrupted by the undercurrent of anxiety that used to keep me awake. I woke up feeling refreshed, with a newfound vitality that carried me through the day. Emotionally and psychologically, the transformation was even more striking. The constant undercurrent of stress that had become my norm started to recede. I found myself reacting to situations with a newfound calmness and clarity. The overwhelming emotions that used to dictate my responses gave way to a more balanced and grounded perspective. This shift had a ripple effect on all aspects of my life. My relationships, both personal and professional, improved dramatically. I became more present and attentive, able to listen and connect with others on a deeper level. The improved mental clarity and focus enhanced my performance at work, leading to more fulfilling and productive days. Decision-making, which used to be a source of anxiety, became more intuitive and grounded.

Perhaps most importantly, I rediscovered joy in the small, everyday moments – the warmth of the sun on my skin, the laughter of a loved one, the simple pleasure of a quiet moment. These were not new experiences, but my ability to be fully present and appreciate them was a gift that somatic therapy had given me. This journey reshaped my entire being.

Through my personal experience with somatic therapy, I realized the power and potential of this approach. It inspired me to delve deeper, to extend my research in the field, and ultimately, to create this guide and workbook. It is a unique blend of classic somatic therapy principles and hands-on workbook activities—a combination I passionately believe is real, tangible change, offering you the power to process, understand, and evolve on your own terms.

My hope is to provide a practical resource that can assist others in beginning their own journey of healing and self-discovery from the comfort of their homes. Therefore, I am deeply grateful that you've chosen this workbook and trust in this path; it means a great deal to me. I understand how valuable your time is, and I'm truly grateful for the moments you are going to spent with this guide.

If you find it helpful, please consider taking a few minutes to leave a review on Amazon. Your feedback not only supports my work but also aids others in discovering this resource, which could be the start of their healing journey.

You can also share your insights and experiences by reaching out directly at **hello@ booksquarepublishing.com,** as well. Your thoughts are extremely important to us, and we are eager to hear what you think!

**I WANT TO WRITE
A REVIEW ON
AMAZON :)**

# UNDERSTANDING SOMATIC THERAPY

Before we dive deeper, let's frame our journey into somatic therapy—a journey that began, for me, with a breakdown. This was a breakdown that, step by painstaking step, illuminated the profound interconnectedness of my physical sensations and emotional state. Through practices like mindful movement, breathwork, and tuning into my body's wisdom, I began to release years of built-up tension. Each step forward in somatic therapy was a step toward uncovering my true self, peeling away layers of stress and trauma that I'd carried for too long. Yes, initially confronting the energy surge linked to past traumas was intimidating, but it also marked the beginning of true healing. Learning to find and use internal resources to soothe myself during intense moments of recollection taught me resilience and self-compassion.

Now, I hear the skeptics who doubt the scientific foundation of somatic therapy, but let me set the record straight. The connections between our bodies and our minds aren't just theories; they're well-documented in neuroscience. Fields as diverse as astrophysics and psychology have contributed to this understanding, with Nobel Prize-winning work by scientists like Kandel shining a light on how deeply interconnected our physical and mental experiences are. This isn't just science; it's a revolution in how we understand the psychology of healing.

Consider the groundbreaking research in the field of psychoneuroimmunology, which investigates the symphony of interactions between our psychological processes, nervous system, and immune system. Take, for instance, the landmark study that revealed how stress can suppress immune function, making us more susceptible to illness. This work has laid the foundation for further explorations into how somatic practices can bolster our immune response. By engaging in mindful movement or therapeutic touch, we are not just easing the tension in our bodies; we're potentially fortifying our defenses against disease. Another pivotal study within psychoneuroimmunology examined the effects of positive emotions on inflammation levels. It was discovered that individuals who engage in practices that promote positive mental states, such as gratitude or compassion exercises—both of which can be integral to somatic therapy—exhibit lower levels of inflammatory biomarkers. This suggests that our emotional landscape is deeply entwined with our physical well-being, and that by nurturing positive feelings, we may also be nurturing our bodies. Moreover, the burgeoning field of epigenetics within psychoneuroimmunology has shown us that our environment and behaviors can influence the way our genes are expressed. Somatic practices, through their impact on our stress levels and emotional states, may influence gene expression in a way that promotes health.

If you're keen to delve into psychoneuroimmunology and explore the pivotal studies that have forged our understanding of the intricate mind-body nexus, let's highlight some significant research that has made substantial contributions. These studies lay the scientific groundwork for therapeutic modalities that seamlessly weave together mental and physical health, including the nuanced practices of somatic therapy.

**Key Contributions in Psychoneuroimmunology:**

- The Pioneer Work of Ader and Cohen: One of the foundational studies in the field was conducted by Robert Ader and Nicholas Cohen in the 1970s. They demonstrated the interaction between the nervous system and the immune response in conditioning experiments with rats, laying the groundwork for the field of psychoneuroimmunology.

- The Impact of Stress on Immune Function: Dr. Sheldon Cohen and colleagues have conducted extensive research on the role of stress in susceptibility to the common cold. His work, particularly a study from the early 1990s, found that people who reported higher stress levels were also more likely to develop a cold when exposed to the virus.

- Positive Emotions and Immune Function: Studies by researchers such as Dr. Barbara Fredrickson and Dr. Sheldon Cohen have examined how positive emotions can enhance immune function. Fredrickson's 'Broaden and Build' theory of positive emotions suggests that these emotions can expand thinking and actions, contributing to improved physiological functioning.

- Mindfulness Meditation and Immune Response: A landmark study by Davidson and colleagues in 2003 found that mindfulness meditation could produce changes in brain activity associated with more positive affect and could also boost immune function, as evidenced by higher influenza antibody titers in participants who meditated.

- The Role of Social Support: A seminal study by Dr. Janice Kiecolt-Glaser and Dr. Ronald Glaser in the 1980s found that medical students who had strong social support had better immune function during exams compared to those with weaker social networks.

The evidence is clear: our bodies listen to our stories, our emotions, and our thoughts, responding in kind with health or illness. We also find rich, anonymized stories that reflect this statement. There's the tale of a woman whose decades-long battle with anxiety began to ease when she discovered the calming cadence of breathwork and mindful movement. Through the somatic therapy process, she learned to navigate her anxiety not just with her mind, but with her body as her ally, transforming her once crippling panic into manageable ripples of concern. Or consider the story of a veteran, grappling with the invisible scars of war, who found in somatic experiences a path to peace that traditional talk therapy couldn't pave. As he learned to listen to the tremors and tensions of his body, he started to piece together a narrative of healing, step by delicate step, moving towards a life where he could once again find solace and joy.

So, these case studies, alongside rigorous research, offer a validation for the somatic journey and the potential that lies within our own forms to heal, grow, and transform, given the right support and guidance. Somatic therapy, therefore, is not just a method or practice but a validated path to wholeness. Somatic therapy stands as a testament to this dialogue, offering practices that whisper to our biology in the language of care, attention, and nurturing. As we engage in this dance of mind and body, we're participating in an age-old conversation, one that science is now articulating with clarity and evidence. It's a powerful affirmation that in healing ourselves, we're not just touching our thoughts or our emotions but influencing the very fabric of our biological being.

Personally, it opened my eyes and my heart to the language of my body, teaching me to listen to its subtle signals and honor its wisdom. For me, this journey wasn't just about healing; it was a transformative experience that reshaped my entire essence, giving me a zest for life and resilience I'd never known. And now, I'm here to guide you through this same journey. As we peel back the layers of trauma, explore the impact on our bodies, and delve into the history and evolution of somatic practices, we embark on a journey of healing and discovery together.

## What is Somatic Therapy?

First and foremost, it's essential to grasp that somatic therapy isn't merely a form of therapy. It's a philosophy, a profound recognition of the intricate connection between our physical existence and our mental and emotional landscapes. It acknowledges our bodies not just as vessels navigating through life, but as repositories for our lived experiences, memories, and traumas.

Consider the nature of trauma: it re-emerges not as clear-cut memories but as visceral reactions, a testament to the fact that trauma bypasses our brain's typical storage for clear narratives, opting instead for a more primal record of images and bodily sensations. This is why the mere act of remembering or encountering reminders of past traumas can evoke such physical responses as chest tightness or stomach knots. These sensations aren't arbitrary but integral components of our emotional experiences, signaling a body that believes it remains under threat.

Hence, the core of somatic therapy lies in tuning into these bodily sensations, listening deeply to what they're attempting to communicate, and unraveling the stories etched beneath our skin. It's about acknowledging that our physical responses are not mere reactions but messages from our deepest selves, urging us to listen and heal.

What sets somatic therapy apart is its commitment to experiential learning. Unlike traditional talk therapies, which often focus on discussing problems to uncover resolutions, somatic therapy invites you to engage directly with your body. It asks you to notice how thoughts, emotions, and experiences manifest physically, using methods like body scanning, movement therapy, and breathwork to navigate the interplay of tension and release within. This approach is not a one-size-fits-all remedy but a deeply personal journey that honors your unique experiences and needs. It melds movement, touch, and mindfulness, offering a holistic path to healing that fosters profound transformations across both physical and emotional realms.

Moreover, somatic therapy ventures beyond mere cognitive restructuring, typical of Cognitive Behavioral Therapy (CBT), to address the physiological roots of stress and anxiety. It employs a 'bottom-up' approach, aiming to recalibrate the autonomic nervous system and facilitate the discharge of trauma. This is in contrast to 'top-down' methods that work primarily through cognitions and behaviors.

Comparisons with therapies like Eye Movement Desensitization and Reprocessing (EMDR) and Cognitive Processing Therapy (CPT) reveal somatic therapy's unique focus on bodily sensations and the experiential aspect of healing. While EMDR and CPT have their strengths, particularly in reprocessing traumatic memories and restructuring trauma-induced thoughts, somatic therapy offers a distinctive path that emphasizes the body's role in healing and resilience.

As we delve deeper into this book, we'll explore the rich history of somatic therapy, its diverse techniques, and how it can help you reconnect with your body, release trapped emotions, and cultivate well-being. It's important to remember, however, that while somatic therapy has wide applicability, it may not be suitable for everyone. Individuals with certain medical conditions or disabilities should approach somatic practices with caution and seek professional advice before beginning.

In summary, somatic therapy offers a unique and holistic approach to healing, one that integrates body, mind, and spirit to navigate the complex aftermath of trauma and stress. Through this journey, you'll discover tools for self-regulation, awareness, and care that can transform your relationship with yourself and the world around you.

## Understanding Trauma and Its Impact

Stepping back into the past, I recall a pivotal moment in my life, a car accident that was both violent and sudden. The sounds of screeching tires, breaking glass, and the palpable air of panic remain etched in my memory. In the aftermath, my nights were haunted by nightmares, my days by flashbacks, and each time I sat behind the wheel, a gripping fear took hold. This experience underscored a profound truth: trauma's effects linger far beyond the healing of physical injuries, embedding themselves deeply within both body and mind.

Trauma manifests in varied forms—physical, emotional, and developmental, each leaving its distinct mark on our beings. The aftermath of significant events, such as accidents or personal losses, is often recognized as traumatic. Yet, it's crucial to acknowledge that trauma doesn't always stem from life-altering occurrences. Sometimes, it's the accumulation of smaller, seemingly inconsequential moments that can unexpectedly overwhelm us. Consider the experience of a young child witnessing a violent argument between parents. While the child may not fully grasp the event's gravity at the moment, the impact on their sense of security can be profound, instilling long-lasting fear and anxiety.

Trauma is not merely an abstract notion but a lived reality that can surface in various ways. Physical and emotional trauma might come barreling into our lives with the force of a storm, or it might be the slow, steady drip of neglect that wears away at our foundations. Symptoms of this upheaval may manifest as a relentless backache, the kind that gnaws at your concentration, or as a heart that races at the mere hint of conflict, a legacy of too many arguments overheard as a child. It can be the insomnia that stretches long nights into infinity or the stomach that churns with a sea of unspoken words and unshed tears.

The spectrum of trauma's expressions is as vast and varied as the human experience:

- Tension headaches that arise like unwelcome visitors
- A pervasive weariness that clings to your limbs, heavy as the evening fog
- An anxiety that flutters in your chest, a trapped bird seeking escape
- Flashbacks that crash over you, unbidden waves of a stormy sea
- Moments of disconnection, when you feel as though you are watching your life from afar, a spectator to your own story

And in developmental trauma, the choreography is intricate and often invisible. It's in the way we might recoil from intimacy, a subconscious echo of trust broken before it could form. It's found in the fierce independence that refuses assistance, a mask for the fear that no one will be there to catch us if we fall. It may lead to a disconnection from one's body, a sense of numbness, or a disassociation from physical sensations, often rooted in early experiences of neglect or abuse. Patterns of chronic tension or discomfort in specific muscle groups can also indicate the body's ongoing efforts to protect itself from perceived threats. Furthermore, developmental trauma can disrupt the nervous system, leading to hypersensitivity to stress, heightened startle responses, and difficulties in achieving relaxation.

In the crucible of healing, we must learn to hold these threads—of loss, of fear, of pain—with care and curiosity. Somatic therapy offers us the tools to do just that: to gently pick apart the knots of our history, to smooth out the creases of our protective armors, and to reweave a narrative of strength and resilience. It's a journey of recognizing how trauma has shaped our bodies and minds, and only by understanding these influences can we pave the way for true healing and transformation.

## Understanging Your Truma

Understanding which trauma is related to our emotional and physical experiences can be complex and requires a nuanced approach. Moreover, trauma can manifest differently in everyone, and what might be traumatic for one person may not be for another. The intensity and impact of trauma can vary greatly from person to person, and events that are traumatic for one individual might not affect another in the same way. The context of the event, the individual's past experiences, support systems, and personal resilience all play critical roles in how trauma manifests and is experienced. Also, understanding that the categorizations can sometimes overlap, as an event could simultaneously impact someone physically and emotionally, is important.

Approach this list with thoughtful consideration; it's here to serve as a guide for reflection, a tool to prompt introspection and aid in identifying possible sources of trauma. Remember, trauma is an individual experience—deeply personal and unique to each person's narrative. I cannot emphasize enough the importance of using this list as a starting point for inquiry, not as a definitive answer. Let it inspire questions and exploration, recognizing that the true understanding of trauma's impact comes from within your personal context and history.

# How to Start Untangling the Threads

### 1. Reflect on Life Events:

- List significant life events, including any known traumatic events, and note any emotional or physical symptoms that arose following these events.
- Consider periods of prolonged stress, even if they didn't result in a specific incident, as these can lead to trauma over time.

### 2. Notice Patterns in Physical Responses:

- Pay attention to when physical symptoms such as pain, tension, or fatigue occur. Do they have any correlation with certain memories, thoughts, or feelings?
- Keep track of your bodily responses in a journal to see if there is a consistent trigger or theme.

### 3. Explore Emotional Reactions:

- Observe your emotional reactions to different situations. Are there disproportionate or intense feelings that seem to be triggered by specific interactions or reminders?
- Consider whether there are underlying fears, anxieties, or beliefs associated with these emotions that might point to past trauma.

### 4. Mind-Body Connection:

- Engage in mindful practices like meditation or yoga to become more attuned to your body's signals and what they might mean.
- Somatic therapies can help you explore the connection between physical sensations and emotional experiences.

### 5. Patterns in Relationships and Behaviors:

- Look at your patterns in relationships. Do you notice repeated dynamics that cause you distress? This could point to developmental trauma.
- Examine your behavior patterns. Do you find yourself engaging in self-sabotage, avoidance, or compulsive behaviors? These could be protective mechanisms developed in response to trauma.

### 6. Professional Guidance:

- A mental health professional, particularly those trained in trauma-informed care, can help you explore your history and symptoms to identify the roots of trauma.
- Therapists can use various assessments and therapeutic interventions to help uncover and understand trauma, such as narrative therapy, psychodynamic approaches, or body-centered practices.

### 7. Educate Yourself:

- Learn about trauma and its effects. Books, workshops, and reputable online resources can provide valuable information.
- Understanding common responses to trauma, such as the fight, flight, freeze, or fawn responses, can provide insight into your own experiences.

### 8. Safe Exploration:

- Ensure that you explore these areas in a safe and supportive environment, as delving into traumatic memories can be destabilizing.
- Take care not to force memories or connections; understanding trauma can be a gradual process that unfolds over time.

# TYPICAL EVENT

| Physical Trauma | Emotional Trauma | Developmental Trauma |
|---|---|---|
| Accidents (e.g., car accidents, falls, sports injuries) | Bereavement and loss of a loved one | Chronic neglect or unstable caregiving during childhood |
| Surgery and medical interventions | Emotional abuse or neglect | Physical, emotional, or sexual abuse in early life |
| Physical assault or abuse | Witnessing violence or severe distress in others | Growing up in a household with addiction or mental illness |
| Natural disasters (e.g., earthquakes, hurricanes) | Betrayal or abandonment in personal relationships | Bullying or social exclusion during formative years |
| Combat or terrorism-related events | Severe life stressors such as job loss or financial crisis | Witnessing domestic violence or severe discord in the home |

# SYMPTOMS OF TRAUMA

| Physical Trauma | Emotional Trauma | Developmental Trauma |
|---|---|---|
| Chronic pain in muscles and joints | Anxiety and panic attacks | Difficulty forming close relationships |
| Persistent fatigue | Depression or persistent mood swings | Distrust and suspicion in intimate situations |
| Gastrointestinal issues | Emotional numbness or detachment | Low self-esteem or feelings of worthlessness |
| Elevated heart rate or palpitations | Flashbacks and intrusive thoughts | Challenges with body image |
| Difficulty sleeping or disturbances | Fearfulness or paranoia | Impaired emotional regulation |
| Hyperarousal or hypervigilance | Difficulty trusting others | Sensation of chronic emptiness or loneliness |

# ADDRESSING THE SYMPTOMS

| Physical Trauma | Emotional Trauma | Developmental Trauma |
|---|---|---|
| Engage in regular, gentle physical activity like yoga or swimming to alleviate tension. | Seek therapy, such as cognitive-behavioral therapy (CBT) or Eye Movement Desensitization and Reprocessing (EMDR). | Engage in long-term psychotherapy, especially therapies that focus on attachment and relational issues. |
| Explore physical therapies such as massage or acupuncture. | Develop a mindfulness meditation practice to help manage anxiety. | Consider somatic experiencing to reconnect and recalibrate the body's response to stimuli. |
| Practice relaxation techniques and ensure proper rest and nutrition. | Use journaling or creative expression to process emotions. | Establish routines that foster a sense of safety and predictability. |
| Consult healthcare professionals for persistent pain or sleep issues. | Build a support network of friends, family, or support groups. | Work on building trust incrementally through consistent and positive interpersonal experiences. |

## The Science of Trauma and the Body

Imagine it's 9pm, and you're navigating a deserted street when suddenly, the sound of footsteps echoes behind you. Instantly, your heart races, palms sweat, and a surge of adrenaline floods your system. This intense reaction is the embodiment of your body's innate defense mechanism—the fight-or-flight response, a complex ballet of neurobiology and physiology in action.

Our daily emotional experiences are the result of complex biochemical processes, which are typically referred to as the "biochemical basis of emotion" or "neurochemical responses" and involve hormones and neurotransmitters that affect how we feel and respond to stimuli (These intricate systems are the subject of study in neurobiology and psychology, particularly within fields such as affective neuroscience, which explores how neurons and complex neural systems result in emotional experiences). When trauma strikes, be it from an abrupt calamity or a profound personal loss, our stress response jolts awake. The hypothalamus, a sentry at the base of the brain, beckons the adrenal glands to flood our system with cortisol and adrenaline. These are the hormones that prepare us to face danger head-on or to flee to the sanctity of safety, rallying our energy and sharpening our senses for the challenges at hand.

But what of the aftermath, when the danger has passed? For those touched by trauma, the physiological imprint of stress response can become a relentless companion. Their bodies, etched with the memory of past perils, remain in a state of heightened readiness, vigilant to the faintest echo of threat. This perpetual guard can give rise to the restless unease of insomnia, a temper that flares at the slightest provocation, and a startle response as quick as lightning—these are the signatures of post-traumatic stress disorder (PTSD), a shadow that may fall long after the traumatic event.

PTSD, a traveler that often arrives without warning, can set in within months of trauma or delay its visit, making itself known through symptoms that linger and disrupt the rhythm of daily life—symptoms that are not the echoes of substance use or other medical conditions.

In the intricate tapestry of the human brain, trauma stitches its indelible marks across various neural regions. The amygdala, ever the sentinel, stands guard, scanning for threats. When trauma infiltrates our psyche, this vigilant watchtower becomes hypersensitive, poised to sound the clarion call of alarm with even the slightest provocation, turning the world into a landscape rife with perceived threats. Simultaneously, the hippocampus—our memory's scribe—struggles under the weight of stress. Ordinarily a reliable archivist, it begins to falter, and the clarity of our past becomes shrouded in fog. Memories, once crisp and vivid, now fragment into shards, their edges blurring, distorting reality with their broken contours. The narratives we once clung to for our identity and understanding of the world around us become unreliable, muddied by the ripples of trauma. Meanwhile, the prefrontal cortex—the executive of our neural command center, responsible for judgement and decision-making—finds itself beleaguered. In the wake of a hyperreactive amygdala, its once clear and commanding voice is drowned out. The result is akin to trying to find direction in a storm; the calm, rational decisions we seek to make are buffeted by emotional gales, leaving us to navigate without our usual compass.

This turmoil is mirrored in our body's physiological response. Stress responses, inherently designed as temporary measures to ensure survival, can morph into persistent states. Cortisol, the hormone summoned to manage our energy stores and respond to stress, can become a relentless presence when its services are retained too long. Like an army that has overstayed its welcome, it begins to exhaust the very resources it was meant to safeguard, leading to weariness and an increased vulnerability to further stress. Adrenaline, our body's swift mobilizer, meant for quick bursts of action in the face of immediate danger, can also turn into a taxing force. Its continuous flow through our veins can shift from life-saving to life-depleting, draining our strength and vitality, leaving us emptied of the vigor we need to face our daily lives.

The journey to mend the wear and tear of trauma on our minds and bodies is a delicate dance of recovery and balance, a process of soothing the overwrought amygdala, clarifying the fogged memories of the hippocampus, and restoring the measured wisdom of the prefrontal cortex. It's about recalibrating the stress response, welcoming the cortisol and adrenaline back into their roles as occasional allies rather than constant companions. In the realm of healing, we seek to stitch new patterns over the old, to find calm amidst the chaos, and to reclaim the power to respond to our world with intention and peace.

In somatic healing, we can learn to calm the amygdala's alarms, clear the fog in the hippocampus, and restore the pre-frontal cortex's guiding light. It's about recalibrating the stress response, welcoming the cortisol and adrenaline back into their roles as occasional allies rather than constant companions.

In healing, we seek to stitch new patterns over the old, to find calm amidst the chaos, and to reclaim the power to respond to our world with intention and peace. This is the promise held within our own biology—a chance for renewal and peace, a chance to return home to ourselves after the storm of trauma.

## The Therapist Role

A trauma-informed therapist is someone who approaches your experiences with a profound reverence for the ways they've shaped you. They understand that trauma can echo through the body and mind, creating ripples that touch every part of your life. With gentle expertise, they help you feel safe to explore these echoes, validating your feelings, and empowering you to take charge of your healing narrative.

Creating a space where vulnerability is not only allowed but welcomed is the very heartbeat of the therapeutic journey, especially when it's the body's stories we're learning to read. A somatic therapist's role, then, is to hold that space with as much care as one holds a bird with a wounded wing—gently, so as not to startle it into flight. In this space, empathy and acceptance are as crucial as the air we breathe, helping to foster trust and allowing vulnerability to surface. It's about crafting an atmosphere where you feel seen and heard, an environment that is as comforting as a trusted friend's embrace. Here, active listening and a compassionate presence are the foundations upon which the journey of healing is built.

A somatic therapist brings to the table not just skills, but a heart wide open, ready to guide you through the complex tapestry of your experiences with unwavering support and empathy. They're the compass in the sometimes disorienting exploration of your inner landscape, adapting their approach to suit the unique paths you tread. It's a partnership where you're encouraged to take the lead, with the therapist by your side, offering insights and tools to help you rediscover your balance and your strength.

The tools and techniques of somatic therapy are as varied and rich as the history from which they draw. Your therapist might invite you to move, to feel, to express through the arts—each technique a thread that weaves into your self-awareness and healing journey. This isn't just about unraveling the knots of trauma; it's about reknitting them into a pattern of resilience and understanding.

Somatic therapy plants the seeds of resilience deep within you, nurturing them with self-compassion and care until they grow into a steadfast presence that can weather life's storms. Your therapist is there to water these seeds, shining light on your inherent strengths, and teaching you to care for them yourself. It's not just about bouncing back; it's about growing up and out, like branches reaching for the sun, ready to face whatever the skies may bring.

In this place of safety and support, you'll find not just healing, but a wellspring of resilience that will carry you through the ebbs and flows of life. And as you journey through somatic therapy, you learn that every breath, every move, every moment is a step towards a more empowered, more vibrant, more wholehearted you.

## History and Evolution of Somatic Practices

Somatic therapy, with its rich tapestry of wisdom and healing, extends roots far deeper than modern science can trace. It draws from the holistic traditions of ancient Egypt, where the seamless interweaving of the spiritual and physical was essential to wellbeing, and from the Eastern philosophies that view the body as a vessel of life force and consciousness. These cultural doctrines have long recognized what we continue to rediscover today: that the health of the body is inextricably linked to the vibrancy of the spirit and the resilience of the mind. These cultures taught us that healing isn't about treating symptoms but nurturing the whole person.

Fast forward to the 19th century, a time brimming with curiosity and the courage to question the status quo. It's as if society itself was on the cusp of a great awakening, much like those moments in our own lives when we begin to see the world through a new lens. The pioneers of modern psychology, like Wilhelm Wundt and William James, started to peel back the layers of our consciousness, suggesting that our physical experiences and emotional states are not just passing ships in the night but deeply intertwined forces that shape who we are.

And then, there's the 20th century, a period that feels like a revolution of the human spirit. Thinkers and healers like Wilhelm Reich, Moshe Feldenkrais, and F.M. Alexander didn't just observe the human condition; they immersed themselves in the mysteries of the body and mind, much like diving into deep waters, not to escape the world but to discover its hidden treasures. Their work wasn't just about understanding tension and trauma but about unlocking the doors to healing and transformation. It's as if the world itself was stretching, awakening to the profound unity of body and mind, and in this stretching, new paths for healing and self-discovery unfurled. Imagine a garden burgeoning with an array of healing modalities, each like a unique flower with its own fragrance and beauty. Somatic experiencing, sensorimotor psychotherapy, somatic movement therapy, dance/movement therapy—these were just a few blossoms in a field that grew richer and more diverse by the day. It was a time of exploration and expansion, a period when the therapeutic landscape was forever changed by the emergence of these profound healing practices.

As this flourishing took place, the academic world, ever curious and seeking, turned its gaze toward this budding field. Somatic psychology began to weave its way into the curricula of institutions, heralding a new era of understanding and legitimizing somatic therapy as a vital discipline within the broader psychological tapestry. This wasn't just acknowledgment; it was an embrace, a recognition of the intricate dance between the physical and the ethereal within us.

The ripple of this recognition extended into the halls of hospitals and wellness centers, where somatic therapy was welcomed as a harmonious partner to traditional treatments. Integrative healthcare models began to bloom, intertwining somatic techniques with pharmaceutical and talk therapy interventions, embracing the holistic nature of human health and well-being.

This was a time when the efficacy of somatic therapy, with its compassionate approach to trauma recovery, chronic pain, stress reduction, and personal growth, shone brightly, offering a beacon of hope to those navigating the stormy seas of physical and mental health challenges.

As we stand in the present, looking back on the knowledge and wisdom of the past, we're reminded that somatic therapy is more than a method or a practice; it's a journey back to ourselves. It's about finding the courage to listen deeply to our bodies, to move, to breathe, and to heal in ways that honor our innate wisdom and resilience. Like the ancient practices that understood the sacred interconnection of all things, somatic therapy invites us to embrace our whole selves, with all our imperfections and beauty, as we navigate the challenges and triumphs of being human.

# Integrating Somatic Practices into Your Daily Life

Embarking on the path of somatic wellness is like starting a garden—nurturing growth requires both daily care and the willingness to adjust to the needs of each plant. With commitment and a bit of nurturing, you'll find your garden—your body—flourishing in ways you never imagined.

## Cultivating Daily Rhythms for Somatic Wellness

In weaving somatic wellness into your life, think of your routines as the soil that will nourish your journey. Simple, daily rituals like mindful walking or intentional stretching are like water and sunlight to your garden—they're fundamental to the growth you're seeking. And let's not forget the sustenance of rest and relaxation—like meditation or deep breathing—quiet spaces where your body can unfurl and recover, finding balance in the stillness.

Nourishing your body is about more than just what you eat—it's about embracing whole foods that support your somatic wellness as fully as a rich compost nurtures a garden. Remember, the rhythm of restorative sleep is as essential as the seasons—without it, your garden can't thrive.

## Personalizing Your Somatic Landscape

Your somatic practice should be as unique as you are—no two gardens are the same, after all. It starts with the soil of self-awareness: which parts of your garden need the most care? What practices will serve those areas best? From the rich soil of research, choose the seeds—be they yoga, Feldenkrais, or another practice—that will flourish in the unique terrain of your body.

Give yourself permission to experiment. Like a gardener trying out new plants, explore different techniques, noticing how each one takes root in your body. And when you find what works, tailor it to your needs—let it be the trellis that supports your growth toward the sun.

## Sustaining Your Somatic Garden

Just as a garden can't thrive on a single day's watering, consistency in your somatic practice is key to deep-rooted well-being. Establishing a routine is like setting a watering schedule—it ensures that your garden gets the steady care it needs to bloom.

And don't forget to track the seasons of your growth. Notice the changes, the blossoming of new strength, the shedding of old patterns, and the steady green shoot of progress. Be patient with yourself, and when you hit a patch of rocky soil, remember that growth often happens in the most unexpected places.

## The Grounding of Resilience

Beyond the immediate beauty of your garden, somatic therapy fosters an inner resilience—the deep roots that will sustain you through storms and droughts. With the support of a compassionate guide, your therapist, you're not just tending to the present moment; you're preparing for the future, strengthening the soil of your being with self-compassion and care practices.

As you cultivate your inner garden, you'll find that resilience is the fruit of your labor. Through mindfulness exercises and a nurturing approach to yourself, you'll grow to meet life's complexities not as harsh winds, but as the breezes that teach you to dance.

Embracing the process of somatic wellness is about more than healing—it's about cultivating a garden within that can weather all seasons, a garden that reflects the vibrancy, resilience, and beauty of who you are.

# Foundations of Somatic Healing

Somatic healing didn't just come to be. It follows a particular process which is rooted in several key principles that guide the therapeutic process. These principles encompass a massive understanding of the body-mind connection and how elements such as physical sensations, movements, and awareness can bring about healing and transformation—it is akin to discovering a hidden language within us.

## Somatic Intelligence: Your Body's Inner Wisdom

Envision somatic intelligence as the body's inherent wisdom, a silent, trusted guide fluent in the language of sensation and feeling, guiding you through life's turbulence. It's the instinctive tightening of muscles in times of danger, the goosebumps that rise in awe or during a moment of profound connection, the gut feelings that signal a deeper knowing beyond words. This is the inner voice that advises when to pause and seek rest, and when to press forward with vigor, ensuring that you're aligned with your well-being.

Somatic therapy opens the door to this profound internal compass, offering us the tools to become fluent in the language of our own physiology. It encourages us to listen—to truly listen—to the subtle pulses and rhythms of our body. By tuning into our body's cues, we unlock the healing power within, tapping into the deep wells of knowledge that our physical form holds. This journey is about more than just recognition; it's about embodiment and integration.

In this process, we learn to embrace the elegance of our body's movements, the mystery of its intuitions, and the intention behind its impulses. Our bodies carry stories and wisdom passed down through generations, coded within the very fibers of our being. By understanding these tales and learning from them, we move through the world with a greater sense of groundedness and connection. We engage in a dance with our experiences, allowing the body's intuition to lead, stepping into a rhythm that feels intrinsically right and good.

Somatic intelligence is our body's way of speaking truths, of signaling needs and desires, of protecting and propelling us towards growth. And somatic exercises are the bridge to enhancing it, allowing us to finely tune into our body's deep wisdom. For instance, through mindful movement practices like slow, deliberate stretching or yoga, we begin to recognize the subtle language of comfort and constraint within our bodies. This can manifest as an awareness of how certain muscles hold stress or how particular postures can affect our mood and energy levels.

Progressive muscle relaxation is another somatic exercise that teaches us the contrast between tension and relaxation. By consciously tensing and then releasing different muscle groups, we learn to identify and let go of physical tightness, which often corresponds to emotional stress. Body scanning is a further somatic technique that promotes deep listening to the body. Lying down comfortably, we mentally traverse our body from head to toe, noting sensations and sending breath to areas that feel stuck or numb. This practice not only develops interoceptive awareness but also teaches us about areas of our body that we often neglect or ignore. Breathwork, another cornerstone of somatic exercises, involves controlling our breathing patterns to influence our mental, emotional, and physical state. Practices like deep diaphragmatic breathing not only provide a sense of calm but also signal the body to relax, highlighting the interconnectedness of breath, emotion, and somatic experience.

With regular practice, we not only develop a deeper understanding of our bodily signals and patterns but also gain the ability to regulate our physiological and emotional responses. This heightened sense of body awareness brings about a greater capacity for self-care and emotional regulation, equipping us with the internal tools needed for healing and resilience. Somatic intelligence thus developed can transform our everyday experience, leading to more mindful, intentional living where the wisdom of the body is recognized, honored, and followed.

## Interoception: The Inner Sensory Experience

Interoception invites us into a deeper relationship with our internal states, from the rhythm of our heartbeat to the flutter of nervousness in our stomach. It's the art of tuning in to our body's unique signals—recognizing the rapid dance of our pulse when excitement takes hold, or feeling the tumultuous churn of our gut as anxiety lurks nearby. This inner sensory experience is a direct line to the ebb and flow of our emotional state, a gauge for the internal climate that influences our reactions and interactions with the world around us.

Somatic therapy serves as a guide, sharpening our perception of these inner cues. It teaches us to discern the subtleties of our body's language, like understanding that a knot in the stomach may signal a need to step back and breathe, acknowledging that it's not just discomfort but a signpost of stress needing attention. For example, when we feel that familiar flutter in our belly before a crucial meeting, we're alerted not just to nerves but to an opportunity to engage in self-soothing strategies—perhaps deep breathing or visualization—to recalibrate and reclaim a sense of calm. When your shoulders tighten, it's as if your body is saying, "Hey, something's weighing on us." Or when your jaw clenches, it's not just tension; it's a silent roar of frustration. Then there's that open, expansive feeling in your chest that comes with a bout of laughter or a moment of pride—it's your heart speaking in its language of joy. Similarly, a racing heart might sweep us into a moment of joy or plunge us into panic.

Through the practice of interoception, we can pause and ask, "What's at the heart of this beat? Is it the thrill of a challenge, or the dread of an anticipated fear?" With this knowledge, we can regulate our response, choosing to ride the wave of exhilaration with grace or to confront fear with grounding techniques that bring us back to a state of equilibrium.

Think about a body scan, like a soft beam of awareness sliding down from the crown of your head to the tips of your toes. It's not a checklist or a task; it's a gentle tour through the home of your soul, your body. You're learning the landscape, the hills and valleys of tension and relaxation, the tight spots that speak of stories untold, and the open spaces that breathe with freedom. And when you take a deep breath, it's about more than just air filling your lungs; it's a message of space and calm to your body. It's like you're telling yourself, "It's okay. I'm here. I'm listening." This is how you start to dance with your emotions, not stepping on each other's toes but moving gracefully, in sync. There's also this magical thing called guided visualization, where you picture a place so safe and serene that just thinking about it makes your muscles loosen, your heart quiet down, and your breath deepen. It's not just imagination; it's your body taking a vacation to this peaceful corner of your mind and soaking up the serenity. Or consider those moments when an emotion sweeps over you—stop and ask yourself, "Where do I feel this? What's the texture of this feeling? Is it sharp like fear or warm like love?" That's you mapping out the terrain of your inner world, understanding the landmarks of your emotions in the physical space of your body.

The whole point of tuning into these whispers of our body with somatic therapy is to learn how to turn them into conversations. Conversations that don't just happen to us but ones we actively engage in. That way, when life turns up the volume and the feelings get intense, we're not swept away. We have the skills to answer back, to soothe and settle ourselves, because we've been listening all along, and we understand the language of our body.

## Body Awareness: The Gateway to Mindful Presence

Body awareness is the quiet hero of our inner narrative, the key that unlocks the door to a more mindful and present existence. Imagine it as a map that shows not just where we are, but also where we've been and where the tension in our muscles wants to take us next. It's in this deepened state of awareness that we can notice how our posture—maybe the curve of a slouch or the collapse of our shoulders—doesn't just speak to our physical state but reflects the weight of our thoughts and the shade of our moods. It's as if our bodies are whispering the stories of our lives, moment to moment, breath to breath.

Let's say you're walking through your day with your shoulders hunched forward, your gaze downward—your entire stance is a message, a signal of how you're engaging with the world. Then, when you consciously straighten up, lift your head, and open your chest, you're not just altering your silhouette; you're inviting a shift in your mental landscape. It's a subtle invitation to the self, suggesting a brighter mood, a more confident outlook. Your body speaks, and your emotions listen, echoing back a change that might have started with a simple stretch or a deep, grounding breath.

But the dialogue doesn't end there. Sometimes, a certain way you hold your hands, or the angle at which you tilt your head, can evoke a memory, a rush of emotion that seems to come from nowhere and everywhere at once. These are the echoes of body memory, where emotions and experiences are etched into our physical form. A scent, a sound, or a touch can pull forward a feeling from this bodily archive, reminding us that we carry our histories not just in our minds but on our skin, in our muscles, in the very way we breathe.

Developing a conscious connection with one's body is akin to learning a new language—the language of self. It's a dialect spoken through tension and ease, through the dance of our diaphragm and the rhythm of our pulse. And as we become fluent, we find that we can not only hear but also respond to our body's needs with more compassion and precision. We learn that a simple act of reaching upward in a morning stretch can be a greeting to the day, a way of telling ourselves, "I am here, I am alive, and I am ready."

In this way, body awareness paves the road to better health and emotional well-being. It invites us to live in conversation with ourselves, where each sensation is a word, each movement a sentence, and each moment of mindfulness a story of who we are becoming. As we walk this bridge of awareness, we discover that every step, every breath, every mindful moment is a step toward a more integrated, healthy, and harmonious life.

## Grounding: Rooted in Stability and Presence

Grounding is our psychological bedrock, the steadying force that whispers through the chaos, "Here I am, and here you stand." It's the practice that brings us back when the world spins too fast, the anchor we drop into the moment that says, "I am safe." Consider the art of mindful walking, where each step becomes a conscious decision, a deliberate communion with the earth beneath our feet. As we walk, we become cartographers of our internal landscape, noting the places where tension resides and using the rhythm of our steps to massage it away, to find that solid place within us that knows how to withstand the storms.

Visualization techniques further cultivate this rootedness, providing not just a mental image but a felt sense. Imagine, for a moment, the sensation of roots extending from the soles of your feet, delving into the rich soil of the earth, tapping into an ancient stability that has long existed before us and will continue long after. It's as if with every mental image of roots burrowing deeper, we are drawing up strength, siphoning calm from the earth's core to fortify our spirit.

This is not just fanciful imagery; it's a profound psychological strategy that leverages the mind-body connection. As we envision these roots, our breathing naturally deepens, our shoulders relax, and our heart rate slows. We become like the oak, whose roots are as expansive below as its branches are above, mirroring the inner work that supports the outer action. We can stand amidst life's unpredictability not as rigid, unyielding entities, but as beings that bend and sway with an inner assurance that we won't be uprooted.

Practices such as these bring us back to our bodies, reminding us of the solidity beneath our feet, the rhythm of our breath, and the capacity within us to endure. They teach us to move through the world with a sense of presence and groundedness that can transform the way we experience everything from everyday stress to profound upheaval. Grounding, therefore, becomes more than a practice—it's a return to ourselves, an affirmation of our resilience, and a promise that no matter what happens, we have the tools to remain centered and steadfast.

## Pendulation: Navigating Between Activation and Relaxation

Pendulation, in the landscape of healing, is akin to a dance—a tender, respectful negotiation with the self, balancing between stillness and motion, holding and releasing. It's the therapeutic embodiment of the ocean's waves: it offers a gentle, rhythmic journey between states of relaxation and activation, allowing for the compassionate exploration of traumatic memories within a safe therapeutic space. This process mirrors the natural ebb and flow of our emotional tides, guiding us toward the release of stored tensions and the integration of past experiences into our narrative of self.

Imagine a scenario where the room feels like a cocoon, safe and soft, and the therapist's voice is a gentle metronome of safety. There, the client is invited to the pendulum swing of healing: to tense, just so, and then, like releasing a breath you didn't know you were holding, to let go. The therapist might say, "Notice the grip in your shoulders—the way they rise towards your ears in remembrance of that old, familiar stress. Now, let's breathe through that tightness, and on an exhale, feel the release, the dropping of weight you've carried far too long."

In this space, the client learns to touch the edges of tension, to feel the shape and contours of stress. They learn to recognize the tightening of muscles, perhaps a subconscious bracing for an impact that lives only in memory. And just as important, they learn to notice the release, the physical sensation of letting go, which might feel as foreign as it does freeing. Each cycle of tension and relaxation, guided by the therapist's experienced, becomes a step on the path back to themselves, a path that acknowledges the trauma but isn't defined by it.

Through pendulation, clients are encouraged to navigate the landscape of their body's responses, to become cartographers of their internal world, mapping where the tension lies and where the peace flows. This process is not about erasing the past but about integrating it, allowing for healing that acknowledges and honors the full story of self. It's a journey that teaches the rhythm of resilience—the ability to move with and through trauma, to let it shape but not control, to acknowledge its presence but also to find release and solace in the here and now.

## Titration: Healing in Manageable Doses

Imagine for a moment you're holding a teacup. If you were to pour in tea too quickly, it would overflow, spilling warmth and water over the edges. That's much like our minds and bodies when facing trauma. The teacup is our capacity to hold and the tea is our traumatic memory. This is where titration comes in, the measured pouring of experience and recollection, ensuring we don't overwhelm our capacity to cope.

In the safe space of a therapist's office, a client—let's call her Emma—sits with clenched fists and breath held tight. She's poised on the edge of a memory, one that's shadowed her steps and stolen her peace. Her therapist, a gentle guide attuned to the subtleties of human emotion, begins the process of titration. They've built a relationship of trust, a shared understanding that Emma's well-being is the beacon they're steering by. Together, they start with the smallest sip of recollection, a mere whisper of the event. Emma mentions the sound of a door slamming from her past, the sharp snap that once heralded a storm of anger in her childhood home. She feels her stomach clench, her heart race. The therapist notices, pausing the narrative, and together they turn towards that sensation. "Let's breathe into that tightness," the therapist encourages, "and find the space around it." As Emma breathes, she imagines space in her body, a buffer between her and the memory. She pictures her feet on the ground, roots growing deep and wide into the earth—her place of safety. The therapist's voice is a lifeline back to the present, a reminder that she's here, not there; safe, not threatened. Emma's breath deepens, her fists unclench, and together they mark this moment of successful navigation through turbulent emotional waters.

The session is a sequence of such moments, a delicate balance between approaching and retreating, a therapeutic rhythm that honors Emma's pace. It's not about reliving the trauma but about acknowledging its shape and weight in her life, and learning to carry it without buckling. Through titration, Emma learns that she can touch her pain without being consumed by it, and in this realization, lies the path to her healing.

## Sequencing: Unraveling Patterns of Tension

Let's step into the world of sequencing, an intuitive map that charts the rise and fall of our body's stories. It's akin to tracing the origins of a river, understanding how each tributary of tension and release shapes the course of our well-being. In somatic therapy, we become explorers of our own internal landscapes, paying attention to the sequences in which our body responds to the world around us.

Consider a client, Julia, who walks into her therapist's office carrying the weight of recurring tension headaches. Each session becomes a journey of tracing these headaches back to their source, much like following the breadcrumbs in a fairytale forest. The therapist encourages Julia to become an attentive observer of her own body, to notice the muscle tightening across her shoulders as she recounts a recent argument with a loved one; to feel the way her jaw clenches when she speaks of unmet expectations at work. As Julia shares her experiences, she and her therapist begin to sketch a map of her physical reactions, charting the course of tension as it travels and transforms. Julia notices that the tension begins as a tightness in her shoulders, a physical manifestation of carrying emotional burdens, before it creeps up, winding its way to the base of her skull, escalating into a full-blown headache.

Through the practice of sequencing, Julia learns to anticipate the onset of this tension. With her therapist's guidance, she starts to recognize the early signs and employs strategies to address them—maybe it's stepping away for a moment of solitude, practicing deep neck stretches, or writing down her feelings to process them more constructively.

This process isn't just about alleviating physical discomfort; it's about unraveling the threads of Julia's somatic narrative to understand the story her body is telling. It's a tale of how emotional stress and unresolved conflicts manifest physically, and how by listening and responding to these signals, Julia can write a new chapter—one of awareness, healing, and resolution.

## Resourcing: Drawing Strength from Within

Resourcing empowers us to tap into our internal reservoirs of strength and resilience, calling upon positive memories, relationships, and qualities that foster feelings of security and well-being. These resources act as anchors, helping us navigate through moments of distress with a renewed sense of support and stability. It is like gathering stones to build a sturdy hearth, a personal sanctuary where we can rekindle our inner flame, even when the winds of life howl fiercely around us. It's an art, really—the art of recognizing and harnessing the vast array of personal and environmental resources that weave through our lives. These are the elements that, when called upon, provide warmth and light in the moments of existence.

Take Michael, for instance, who faces the ups and down of daily pressures. When the tide rises, and the stresses of life threaten to engulf him, he reaches for the stones he's gathered over time. There's the smooth one, etched with the memory of a sunlit beach—the place of solace where the only deadlines were the receding tides. There's the speckled one, symbolizing his trusty companion, Sam, whose easy laughter can cut through the thickest tension. And then there's the solid one, representing his deep love for painting, where every stroke is a conversation between color and canvas, a dialogue that drowns out the clamor of worries. Each stone, each resource, is a testament to Michael's ability to withstand and adapt. When anxiety's shadow looms, he pulls these stones close, feeling their weight and texture, grounding himself in their reliability. A mental journey back to the beach lowers his heart rate, a phone call to Sam reignites his optimism, and an hour with his paints restores his sense of control.

Somatic therapy guided Michael in gathering these stones, teaching him to notice which memories fortified his spirit, which relationships served as lifelines, and which activities replenished his strength. Now, as he navigates life's complexities, he has a wellspring of resources to draw from. In times of challenge, he's not merely surviving; he's supported by a network of emotional buttresses, each resource a beacon reminding him of his capacity for resilience, his potential for growth, and the indelible strength that lies within.

# Somatic Movements

Embarking on the exploration of traditional practices, we dive into a world where movement and mindfulness interlace, carrying with them ancient wisdom that holds secrets of balance, connection, and holistic well-being. Each of the follwing traditional practices—yoga, qigong, tai chi, aikido, Pilates, and dance—serves as a lighthouse. They remind us that within the rhythm of movement and the silence of stillness lies the key to our well-being. As we delve into these ancient arts, we discover that the journey to balance and harmony is not just a path we walk, but a dance we live.

## Yoga: A Dance of Breath and Movement

Yoga, with its roots burrowed deep into ancient far East Indian soil, emerges as a beacon of holistic health, addressing the physical, mental, and spiritual dimensions of our being. It's a practice that unfolds on the mat as a series of postures, breathwork, and meditation, yet its essence transcends far beyond, touching the very core of our existence. Yoga beckons us to a place of inner stillness amidst the chaos, where the harmony between mind, body, and spirit illuminates the path to enlightenment. For those who may not tread the spiritual path, yoga still offers a sanctuary—a haven of flexibility, strength, and tranquility. Its diverse styles ensure that, whether you seek the gentle flow of Hatha or the vigorous rhythms of Vinyasa, there's a place for you in yoga's embrace, promising a journey toward physical and mental clarity.

**Benefits:** Yoga promotes flexibility, muscle strength, and stress reduction. It enhances respiratory endurance and cardiovascular health, improves posture, and fosters a deep sense of inner peace.

**Challenges/Contraindications:** Some yoga poses can be challenging for individuals with joint issues or chronic pain. It's important to start with appropriate levels and consult with a professional, especially if there are concerns like high blood pressure or pregnancy.

## Qigong and Tai Chi: The Art of Flow

In the graceful dance of Qigong and Tai Chi, we find the ancient Chinese secrets to vitality and serenity. These practices, akin to moving meditation, cultivate the flow of qi—life energy—through gentle movements and conscious breath. Accessible to all ages, it's a harmonious ballet of mind, body, and spirit, where each gesture is a stroke of energy, painting tranquility across the canvas of our being. These practices whisper of stress relief, flexibility, and mental clarity, inviting us into a world where health and inner peace flourish.

**Benefits:** These practices increase joint flexibility and stability, improve balance and proprioceptive skills, and decrease stress. They're also associated with better immune function and lowered blood pressure.

**Challenges/Contraindications:** While generally low-impact, this practices may require caution for those with balance issues. Overdoing certain movements can lead to muscle strain, so it's crucial to maintain proper form.

## Aikido: The Way of Harmony

Aikido, a jewel in the crown of Japanese martial arts, teaches us the art of peace—a path where harmony with an opponent's energy leads to balance and control. This practice of circular movements and joint locks is more than self-defense; it's a philosophy woven into the fabric of our daily encounters. Aikido cultivates a way of being that embraces compassion, resilience, and ethical integrity, guiding us to navigate life's conflicts with grace and inner strength.

**Benefits:** Aikido offers a full-body workout that improves flexibility, coordination, and reflexes while also instilling principles of peace and conflict resolution.

**Challenges/Contraindications:** The dynamic throws and falls require careful practice and may not be suitable for individuals with severe osteoporosis or those with a high risk of fractures.

## Pilates: Sculpting Strength from Within

Pilates emerges from the early 20th century as a symphony of movement designed to strengthen, align, and rejuvenate. Its precise, controlled exercises—a blend of strength and flexibility—echo the profound connection between mind and body, inviting mindfulness into every motion. Pilates stands as a testament to the power of self-awareness in shaping our physical health, offering a path to poise and vitality for everyone.

**Benefits:** Pilates is celebrated for core strengthening, improved posture, and alignment. It enhances muscle control and can aid in rehabilitation after injuries.

**Challenges/Contraindications:** Certain Pilates exercises may need to be modified for those with lower back pain or neck issues. It's vital to ensure movements are done with proper technique to avoid injury.

## Dance: The Soul's Expression

Within the realm of dance, from the spontaneity of Contact Improvisation to the explorative journey of Ecstatic Dance we uncover the layers of our being. Dance becomes a mirror reflecting our deepest selves, a space where movement and emotion intertwine, revealing truths hidden in the rhythm of our bodies. It invites us to play, to explore, and to connect—transforming the dance floor into a canvas of personal discovery and expression.

**Benefits:** Dance boosts cardiovascular health, increases stamina, improves balance and coordination, and uplifts mood. It's a creative outlet that encourages emotional expression and connection with others.

**Challenges/Contraindications:** High-impact or vigorous dance styles might pose risks to those with joint problems or cardiovascular issues. It's important to choose a style and intensity level that matches one's fitness and health status.

I highly encourage you to download the bonus material and explore the exhilarating world of **Ecstatic Dance**. This unique form of expression allows you to move freely without any structured steps or routines, helping you connect deeply with yourself as you flow with the music. To get started, simply play the accompanying music, let go of any inhibitions, and allow your body to move instinctively. Give it a try and feel the transformative impact it can have on your well-being!

# SOMATIC APPROACHES IN ALTERNATIVE MEDICINE

In the world of alternative medicine, we find not just methods of healing but pathways to a deeper communion with ourselves. Each of the following practice, with its unique focus and methodology, offers a lens through which to view the body not as a machine to be fixed, but as a garden to be tended, where every movement and breath can cultivate the ground for growth, transformation, and renewal. However, when we place these practices side-by-side with somatic therapy, we observe a shared reverence for the body's innate intelligence but a divergence in approach. While somatic therapy often directly addresses trauma through body awareness and emotional release, the methods described above may focus more on gradual movement reeducation or energetic balancing. One might choose the Alexander Technique or Feldenkrais for subtle postural adjustments and enhanced self-awareness, Structural Integration for comprehensive bodily alignment, or the Trager Approach for its unique combination of touch and movement, depending on individual needs and healing journeys. I suggest you to embark on any of these paths begins with selecting a practitioner who resonates with your personal healing philosophy. Look for someone with not just credentials but a presence that makes you feel seen and heard. Your initial session should be a dialogue—a space where your history, hopes, and concerns are met with expertise and empathy. Expect to be guided, but also to participate actively in your journey toward wellness. Remember, the goal is not just to heal but to flourish within the embrace of these time-honored practices.

## The Alexander Technique: Unwinding the Threads of Tension

The Alexander Technique emerges as a beacon of mindful movement, illuminating the subtle ways our habitual tensions shadow our natural posture and grace. Developed by Frederick Matthias Alexander, this method gently coaxes us to shed these layers of strain, inviting a renaissance of movement that is both freer and more aligned. Imagine each session as a journey back to your body's original blueprint, where movement is not just about reaching from point A to B but about rediscovering the joy of unencumbered motion. This technique doesn't just teach us how to move; it teaches us how to live with ease, turning every step and gesture into a reflection of our newfound balance and poise.

**Benefits:** The Alexander Technique can lead to improved posture, reduced muscle tension, and greater ease in movement. It often results in better stress management and can contribute to pain relief, especially for chronic conditions related to misalignment and tension.

**Challenges/Contraindications:** Those with certain musculoskeletal issues should approach the Alexander Technique carefully and preferably under the guidance of a healthcare provider. Additionally, because it requires a degree of self-reflection and proprioceptive awareness, it may initially be challenging for individuals who are not used to introspective practices.

## The Feldenkrais Method: The Art of Somatic Exploration

The Feldenkrais Method stands as a testament to the profound wisdom of the body, offering a mosaic of movements that invite us to explore the boundaries of our physical and mental landscapes. With Moshé Feldenkrais at the helm, this approach weaves together a tapestry of gentle motions and attentive awareness, prompting an intimate dialogue with the self. It's as if each movement is a question posed to the body, and in its response, we find the keys to unlock patterns of tension and rediscover the fluidity of motion that is our birthright. This method is not just about moving better; it's about a deeper connection to the self and a more harmonious way of being in the world.

**Benefits:** The Feldenkrais Method can increase self-awareness, improve mobility and flexibility, and enhance neurological functioning. It's particularly helpful for those recovering from injuries as it focuses on gentle movements that can be therapeutic.

**Challenges/Contraindications:** It may not be suitable for individuals with severe mobility restrictions or those who require a more active form of therapy. It's also a practice that demands mental engagement, which can be a barrier for those looking for a more passive treatment modality.

## Structural Integration: Sculpting the Body's Resilience

Within the realm of Structural Integration, including Rolfing and Hellerwork, lies a sculptural approach to bodywork that seeks to mold our structure into its most efficient and aligned form. This practice delves into the body's fascial web, seeking out areas of imbalance and restriction to release and realign. It's a process that mirrors the natural forces of gravity and levity, grounding us firmly to the earth while lifting us toward our fullest potential. Through hands-on manipulation and movement education, Structural Integration reeducates the body and mind, inviting a transformation that can be as profound as it is palpable. It's a journey toward feeling more at home in our own skin, moving with grace and living with ease.

**Benefits:** This method is excellent for addressing posture issues, chronic pain, and improving overall body alignment. It's known to enhance physical performance and can significantly impact the body's structural integrity.

**Challenges/Contraindications:** Due to its physical intensity, individuals with acute injuries, inflammatory conditions, or those who have recently had surgery should avoid this practice until they have sufficiently healed.

## The Trager Approach: Cultivating Lightness and Ease

The Trager Approach beckons us to discover the lightness of being that comes when we release the physical and mental knots that bind us. Developed by Dr. Milton Trager, this method infuses the therapeutic touch with a sense of exploration and play, encouraging the body to remember states of deep relaxation and fluidity. Through the dance of Mentastics and the nurturing touch of the practitioner, we're invited to explore new landscapes of movement and sensation, finding freedom from the constraints of habituated tension. The Trager Approach teaches us that within every movement, there's an opportunity for joy and liberation, a chance to embody the essence of ease.

**Benefits:** The Trager Approach is effective in releasing deep-seated physical and mental tension, promoting relaxation, and improving mental clarity and physical agility.

**Challenges/Contraindications:** This approach may not be appropriate for those with certain psychological conditions that make touch-based therapies challenging, or for those who have specific pain syndromes where gentle movement may exacerbate symptoms.

# THE PILLARS OF EMBODIED PRESENCE

## Building Body Awareness

In the heart of somatic therapy lies the practice of building body awareness. As we already discuss, it's about learning the language of your body, listening to its silent murmurs and its loud cries, and honoring the stories it tells.

For those eager to cultivate this connection, consider incorporating simple daily practices tailored to your unique capabilities and lifestyle. Whether it's mindful stretching upon waking, intentional pauses throughout the day to check in with your body's posture and sensations, or ending the day with reflective journaling on the body's messages, each act builds the bridge to deeper awareness.

Self-discovery requires us to blend the wisdom of our minds with the innate knowledge of our bodies. It is in the synthesis of mindfulness with body awareness that we discover the full spectrum of our human experience, enhancing not just our perception of the present moment but also our connection to our own physical existence. This integration is essential because it allows us to live in a state of full engagement, where every sense is alive and every emotion is acknowledged and appreciated. It transforms our daily experiences, enabling us to move through the world with a deepened awareness that enriches every interaction and every thought. To effortlessly interlace mindfulness with body awareness, begin with grounding exercises such as focusing on the feeling of your feet in contact with the ground beneath as you walk, which roots you firmly in the now. Savour each bite when you eat, immersing all your senses in the act, and thus making the mundane sacred. Before reacting to stress, pause mindfully; notice the messages your body sends, and respond with intentionality, using breath as a tool to bridge the gap between mind and body. This creates a balanced state, harmonizing the physical with the emotional.

## 1. Recognizing Bodily Signals: Tuning In

Think of your body as a wise old friend, constantly chattering away, eager to tell you how it's feeling—whether it's through a quickened pulse, a tightness in the shoulders, or a warmth in the heart. Tuning into these signals is about pausing in the midst of our chaotic days to really notice these messages. It's about finding stillness in the middle of the storm to hear what's going on inside. By turning our attention to where these sensations bubble up—be it the tension in your jaw or the fluttering in your stomach—we start to piece together a map of our inner landscapes. It's about becoming a detective in your own life, tracing back from the sensation to the emotion or experience that may have sparked it. It's akin to unraveling a ball of yarn, following the thread back to the beginning, understanding the why behind the what.

## 2. Interpreting Bodily Signals: Deciphering the Code

Once we've spotted these signals, the next step is to interpret them, to understand the language of our inner workings. It's like sitting across from a friend who speaks in metaphors and figuring out what they really mean. Is the tightness in your chest a sign of anxiety, or is it anticipation? Is the ache in your back just fatigue, or is it a burden you've been carrying too long? This is not always easy—it's a process that asks for patience and an open heart. It requires us to look at our feelings in the mirror and really see them, maybe for the first time. To ask ourselves, "What's going on here?" and to be ready for the answers. It's about connecting the dots between our physical sensations and our emotional world, crafting a deeper understanding of the interplay between our mind and body.

## 3. Cultivating Mindful Awareness: Becoming Present

Mindful awareness is like a soft, steady light we shine on ourselves, illuminating our experiences with kindness and curiosity. It's about learning to live in the moment, to truly be where we are—whether that's sitting at a red light, standing in line for coffee, or feeling the ground beneath our feet as we walk. Mindfulness can be as simple as paying attention to the breath, feeling it come and go, noticing how it ebbs and flows through our bodies. It can be a body scan, a quiet journey from head to toe, greeting each part of ourselves with gentleness. As we practice, we learn to greet each thought, each feeling, each sensation with a nod of acknowledgment, without judgment or hurry.

## 4. Enhancing Self-Regulation: Steering the Ship

Finally, self-regulation is about learning to steer our own ship, even when the seas are rough. It's about having a toolbox of techniques—like deep breathing, muscle relaxation, or visualization—that we can dip into when the waves of stress, anxiety, or pain wash over us. These are our anchors, the things we can rely on to bring us back to a place of calm and control. Deep breathing might seem like a simple thing, but it's a powerful ally. It tells our body, "It's okay, we've got this," slowing everything down and bringing us back to center. Muscle relaxation is another way we can whisper to our bodies, "You can let go now," releasing the tension we hold onto without even realizing it. And visualization—it's our imagination as a resource, painting pictures in our minds of calm, peaceful scenes that soothe and comfort us. It's about using the power of our minds to create a sanctuary within, a safe space we can retreat to whenever the outside world gets too loud or too heavy.

# The Power of Breathing

Whether you're sitting in quiet meditation, moving through a sequence of yoga poses, or simply pausing for a moment of mindfulness amidst a busy day, breath is a constant companion—a reminder of your ability to navigate your inner world with intention and grace.

Throughout the annals of history and across the spectrum of holistic practices, from the ancient yogic pranayamas to the rhythmic breaths of qigong, the act of breathing has been revered as both a life-sustaining force and a tool for healing. It's a thread that runs through time, binding together traditions that span continents and eras, each culture finding its own rhythm in the ebb and flow of inhalation and exhalation.

The act of breathing transcends mere biological function—it's a profound communion between our inner and outer worlds. It's the first act we perform at birth and the last upon leaving this world, a constant companion and a barometer of our well-being. Holistic practitioners through the ages have understood that breath is a bridge to the unseen, the intangible parts of ourselves. It's as if each breath carries with it a whisper of wisdom, a piece of the universe's vast puzzle, offering us a chance to connect with the cosmic dance of life.

In times of old, shamans and healers would employ breath to enter trance states, to heal and to divine. In the rituals of the Amazonian tribes, the rhythmic breath is central to connecting with the spirits of nature. In the meditative practices of Buddhist monks, breath is the anchor to the present moment, a practice of mindfulness that brings clarity and enlightenment.

Even today, in the hurried rush of modern life, the resurgence of interest in breathwork for health and stress relief echoes the ancient knowledge that breathing is a powerful ally. It's a reminder that despite technological advances and the complexity of contemporary society, the simple, deliberate act of breathing remains one of the most potent tools we have for self-regulation, for transcending the noise and finding a quiet space within.

Breathing—this most instinctual of acts, one we so often take for granted—is intricately tied to our inner world of emotions. Just think about it: when fear or anxiety grips us, our breaths become shallow and quick, as if our body is preparing to fend off an unseen enemy. In contrast, when we're relaxed, our breath deepens, rolling in and out like gentle waves, signaling to our body that all is well. But here's the profound part: we can consciously change our breathing patterns to influence how we feel. That's right, by taking control of our breath, we can shift from a state of unrest to one of tranquility. Imagine you could flip a switch and move from the high-alert stress of fight-or-flight to the serene repose of rest-and-digest. That's the gift of controlled breathing.

Now, let's talk about how this plays out in practice. In the rich traditions of yoga, pranayama exercises teach us to harness our breath's energy—encouraging long, sustained breaths to invigorate our body or gentle exhalations to promote relaxation. Similarly, the Alexander Technique uses conscious breathing to help release muscle tension, guiding us back to a natural state of alignment and ease. Incorporating these breathing exercises into our daily routines is like having a personal toolkit for emotional regulation. Caught in a moment of tension? A few focused breaths can help melt away stress. Overwhelmed by the day's pace? Slowing down your breath can bring a moment of peace amidst the chaos.

Breathwork, in the context of somatic therapy, is like an intimate conversation with the deepest parts of ourselves—it's profound and revealing. When we engage in breathwork, we are essentially practicing the art of self-regulation. This is akin to learning how to conduct the symphony of our nervous system; we can cue a lullaby to calm the rapid rhythms of stress or anxiety or a or conjure up a spirited allegro to awaken and energize our system. The breath has the unique ability to signal our body to downshift from the sympathetic nervous system's 'fight or flight' mode to the parasympathetic's 'rest and digest' state. It's a tool we carry within us at all times, one we can access to steady our heart rate, lower blood pressure, and usher in a sense of calm. Moreover, breathwork enhances body awareness. As we focus on the rise and fall of our chest or the expansion and contraction of our diaphragm, we become more attuned to the subtle nuances of our bodily functions. This attention can lead to a heightened sense of how stress or relaxation feels within us, teaching us to recognize our body's signals before they become screams for attention. Lastly, breathwork serves as a method to weave together the physical and mental threads of our being. Just as a tapestry is formed from the interlacing of individual threads, our well-being is the intricate interplay of body and mind. By using breath as a tool to affect both, we create a holistic harmony, a balance that resonates through every aspect of our existence. This unity leads to vitality, as our optimized breathing nourishes our cells and cleanses our system, leaving us feeling more alive and present.

So you see, learning breathwork is not just a technique; it's a transformation. As we master our breath, we master our response to the world around us, finding a deeper sense of balance and well-being that ripples through every aspect of our lives. To experience these profound benefits, we can incorporate these essential breathing practices into our daily routines. They are designed not only to foster mindfulness and body awareness but also to aid in managing stress and enhancing emotional well-being.

**1. The Grounding Breath:** Close your eyes and find a comfortable seated position. Feel the weight of your body making contact with the chair or floor. Take a slow, deep breath through your nose, and imagine drawing the breath all the way down to your feet, grounding you to the earth. Hold the breath for a moment, then exhale slowly through your mouth, releasing tension and stress from your body. Repeat this for several cycles, with each breath deepening your sense of connection to the ground beneath you.

**2. The Expansive Breath:** Stand or sit with your spine straight and shoulders relaxed. Inhale deeply, filling your lungs from bottom to top as if filling a glass with water. As you inhale, let your ribs expand outwards, creating space in your chest. Hold the breath for a couple of seconds at the top, and then exhale gently, feeling the ribs come back together, pushing all the air out. This exercise helps to open up the body and create a sense of spaciousness within.

**3. The Centering Breath:** Sit with your back straight and hands resting on your lap. Breathe in slowly and imagine a warm, golden light filling your core, centering your energy. As you exhale, visualize any scattered thoughts or feelings being expelled with your breath. This centering breath is excellent for moments when you need to collect your thoughts and emotions.

**4. The Wave Breath:** Lay down comfortably on your back. Close your eyes, and as you breathe in, imagine a wave of relaxation starting at your toes and moving up through your body to the crown of your head. As you breathe out, imagine the wave traveling back down to your toes, washing away any tension. This visualization promotes a full-body relaxation that can be profoundly soothing.

**5. The Soothing Breath:** In a quiet space, inhale gently through your nose while counting to four, feeling the calmness enter your body. Hold the breath for a count of seven, which encourages a pause in the constant stream of thoughts. Then exhale slowly through the mouth for a count of eight, releasing any discomfort or tightness. This breathing pattern can help to soothe an anxious mind and bring you back to a state of balance.

## Grounding: Anchoring in the Now

Within the swirling tides of our daily lives, grounding techniques stand as pillars—solid, reassuring, and nurturing. They draw us back from the tumult of past regrets and future anxieties, anchoring us firmly in the present moment. These practices are not just about touching base with where we are; they are about rooting ourselves there, feeling the steadiness of the earth beneath our feet, and from that place of stability, finding the clarity and calm to face whatever comes our way.

**1. Mindfulness Meditation:** This practice is an invitation to stillness, a space we create within ourselves to observe the flow of our thoughts and feelings without getting swept away. Mindfulness meditation begins with finding a quiet spot and adopting a comfortable position, whether sitting, lying down, or even walking. We focus on our breath, the inhale and exhale, the rise and fall of our chest, or the air moving through our nostrils. As thoughts intrude—and they will—we acknowledge them like passing clouds in a vast sky, without judgment, and return our focus to the breath. Over time, this practice can build our capacity to remain present and composed, even amidst the storms of life.

**2. Visualization Techniques:** Visualization is a powerful way to connect with the grounding energy of nature, even when we're indoors. It involves closing our eyes and picturing ourselves in a serene natural setting—a forest, a beach, a mountain, or any place that evokes a sense of peace. We engage all our senses: the scent of pine or saltwater, the sound of leaves rustling or waves lapping, the feel of the ground beneath us. By immersing ourselves in this sensory experience, we forge a connection to the natural world that sustains and grounds us.

**3. Nature Connection:** Direct engagement with nature is a deeply grounding practice. Walking barefoot on grass, touching the bark of a tree, or simply sitting and watching the sky can bring us back to the present moment. This connection reminds us that we are part of a larger, living system and helps dissolve the illusion of isolation.

**4. Body Scan:** A body scan is a journey through the body where we pay attention to each part, noticing any sensations of tension, discomfort, or relaxation without trying to change them. Starting from the toes and moving upward, we observe, acknowledge, and breathe into every area of our body. This not only grounds us but can also reveal where we hold our stress and how it affects our physical state.

**5. Focused Tasks:** Engaging in simple, repetitive tasks like knitting, gardening, or even washing dishes can be grounding. The key is to perform these tasks with full attention, observing the movements, the textures, and the sensations involved, allowing the rhythm to bring a sense of calm focus.

**6. Gratitude Exercises:** Taking time each day to note what we're grateful for—a practice known as gratitude journaling—can ground us in the present and foster a positive outlook. By appreciating what we have here and now, we anchor ourselves in the positive aspects of our lives.

# SOMATIC EXERCISES
# FOR TRAUMA SURVIVORS

Somatic exercises are particularly beneficial for trauma survivors because they focus on reconnecting the individual with their body, helping to manage the physical and emotional symptoms of trauma. It's important to approach them gently and with self-compassion, ideally under the guidance of a qualified somatic therapist who can provide support and ensure that these exercises are performed in a safe and therapeutic manner. Each individual's response to trauma is unique, so these exercises may need to be customized to fit personal comfort levels and boundaries.

Here are four sets of somatic exercises that can be especially helpful. These exercises target specific aspects of reconnection and recovery, from grounding and stabilizing to enhancing body awareness and emotional release. For more detailed instructions and to ensure the exercises are aligned with my unique healing process, I can refer to the accompanying PDF exercise sheets.

## Somatic Grounding Exercises

**Earthing:** This involves walking barefoot on natural surfaces like grass, soil, or sand. The direct contact with the earth can help to literally 'ground' a person, allowing them to feel more present and centered.

**Five Senses Exercise:** Engage all five senses one-at-a-time to become fully present. Identify and focus on one thing you can see, hear, touch, taste, and smell.

**Palming:** Rub your hands together until they feel warm, then gently cup them over your closed eyes. Feel the warmth and allow your body to relax, focusing on the darkness and welcoming the calm it brings.

## Breathing Techniques for Regulation

**Diaphragmatic Breathing:** Also known as belly breathing, this technique involves deep breathing that engages the diaphragm, helping to stimulate the parasympathetic nervous system and promote relaxation.

**Extended Exhale:** This technique emphasizes a longer exhale than inhale, which can help calm the nervous system. For instance, inhale for a count of four, then exhale for a count of eight.

**Box Breathing:** Breathe in for a count of four, hold for four, exhale for four, and then hold for four. This pattern can help regulate the nervous system and improve focus.

## Movement and Stretching

**Progressive Muscle Relaxation:** Tense and then release each muscle group in the body, starting from the toes and working up to the top of the head. This helps to release physical tension associated with trauma.

**Yoga Poses:** Certain yoga poses can be particularly beneficial for trauma survivors, such as Child's Pose or Legs Up the Wall, as they promote relaxation and a sense of safety.

**Dance/Movement Therapy:** Engaging in free-form dance or structured movement can help express emotions that may be too difficult to verbalize.

## Interoceptive Awareness Practices

**Body Scan Meditation:** Lie down and mentally scan through each part of your body, observing any sensations without judgment. This practice can increase awareness of physical sensations associated with emotional states.

**Heartbeat Exercise:** Focus on your heartbeat, either by feeling your pulse or simply tuning in to the sensation of your heart in your chest. This can help connect you to your body's rhythm and encourage presence.

**Temperature Awareness:** Holding something warm or cool, such as a cup of tea or a cold stone, and focusing on the sensation can help bring awareness back to the present and away from traumatic memories.

# SELF-ASSESMENT TOOLS

## BODY AWARENESS QUESTIONNAIRE

The BAQ is designed to evaluate how attentively you notice and interpret bodily sensations and signals.

1. I can easily identify when I am feeling tense............................................................SCORE:

2. I notice when my breathing becomes shallow or restricted.................................SCORE:

3. I am aware of changes in my heartbeat without touching my chest....................SCORE:

4. I can recognize signs that indicate I am becoming hungry..................................SCORE:

5. I am conscious of the position of my body while sitting or standing................SCORE:

6. I can detect subtle changes in my body temperature.............................................SCORE:

7. I am aware of sensations in my muscles, such as relaxation or tightness............SCORE:

8. I notice when I start feeling physically tired or fatigued.....................................SCORE:

9. I am aware of minor discomforts in my body, such as slight itching or mild pain........SCORE:

10. I can identify how my body feels in stressful situations.......................................SCORE:

 **How It Works**

Answer the 10 questions on this page.

Use a 1-5 scale for each question where 1 might represent "Never" or "Not at all" and 5 might represent "Always" or "Extremely."

Then, calculate the total scores for all questions.

**TOTAL SCORE**

 **Interpretation**

Scores between 10-20

**Low Body Awareness:** Might benefit from practices that increase body mindfulness, such as yoga or meditation.

Scores between 21-35

**Moderate Body Awareness:** Have a fair sense of body awareness. Might explore deeper practices to enhance this.

Scores above 35

**High Body Awareness:** Have a strong connection with body's sensations. Maintaining or deepening this awareness can be beneficial.

# SELF-ASSESMENT TOOLS

## STRESS RESPONSE SELF-ASSESSMENT

This tool can help you recognize your stress patterns and guide you toward appropriate stress management strategies.

1. I experience physical symptoms like headaches or stomachaches when stressed............SCORE:

2. I find it hard to concentrate or focus on tasks during stressful periods...........................SCORE:

3. I tend to feel irritable or angry under stress.................................................................SCORE:

4. I have trouble sleeping or experience disrupted sleep when I'm stressed.........................SCORE:

5. I often feel anxious or worried when faced with stress....................................................SCORE:

6. I tend to overeat or lose my appetite when I am stressed................................................SCORE:

7. I experience muscle tension, especially in my neck or shoulders, in stressful times.......SCORE:

8. I feel fatigued or drained when I am undergoing stress...................................................SCORE:

9. I tend to withdraw from social interactions or prefer to be alone when stressed...........SCORE:

10. I have noticed an increase in unhealthy habits during stressful periods.......................SCORE:

## How It Works

Answer the 10 questions in this page.

Use a 1-5 scale for each question where 1 might represent "Never" or "Not at all" and 5 might represent "Always" or "Extremely."

Then, calculate the total scores for all questions.

TOTAL SCORE _____

## Interpretation

Scores between 10-20

**Low Stress Response:** Seem to manage stress well. Continue with coping strategies.

Scores between 21-35

**Moderate Stress Response:** Have a fair level of stress response. Mindfulness, relaxation techniques, or lifestyle changes might be beneficial.

Scores above 35

**High Stress Response:** It appears that stress significantly impacts. Consider stress management techniques or professional support.

## SELF-ASSESSMENT AND AWARENESS

## EMOTIONAL WELL-BEING SELF-ASSESMENT

This self-assessment tool helps you reflect on your emotional state and can be a great starting point for understanding your emotional landscape and seeking appropriate support, if needed.

1.  I feel optimistic about the future..................................................................................SCORE:

2.  I feel in control of my emotions...................................................................................SCORE:

3.  I can easily find things to be happy about...................................................................SCORE:

4.  I feel that my life has a sense of purpose....................................................................SCORE:

5.  I am able to bounce back after a hard time.................................................................SCORE:

6.  I feel satisfied with my personal relationships...........................................................SCORE:

7.  I generally feel calm and peaceful...............................................................................SCORE:

8.  I have a good understanding of my feelings and why I feel the way I do....................SCORE:

9.  I am able to express my emotions in a healthy way.....................................................SCORE:

10. I feel a sense of belonging and connection with others..............................................SCORE:

 **How It Works**

Answer the 10 questions on this page.

Use a 1-5 scale for each question where 1 might represent "Never" or "Not at all" and 5 might represent "Always" or "Extremely."

Then, calculate the total scores for all questions.

**TOTAL SCORE**

 **Interpretation**

Scores between 10-20

**Low Emotional Well-being:** It might be helpful to explore areas of life causing distress and seek strategies or support to enhance emotional health.

Scores between 21-35

**Moderate Emotional Well-being:** Have a fair level of emotional health. Identifying and working on areas that challenge emotional well-being could be beneficial.

Scores above 35

**High Emotional Well-being:** Responses suggest good emotional health. Continue with positive habits and emotional coping strategies.

# SELF-ASSESSMENT AND AWARENESS

## EXPLORING MOVEMENT

Exploring movement through both free-form and structured exercises is a dynamic way to enhance body awareness and encourage creativity in movement. Free-form exercises allow for spontaneous, intuitive movements, while structured exercises provide a more guided approach to bodily awareness. This exercise can be practiced regularly, depending on your routine and preference. You might find certain times of the day or week more suitable for free-form or structured movements.

### Objectives

To enhance body awareness and mindfulness through movement.

To encourage creative expression and exploration of movement.

To balance the body and mind with both physical activities.

### Preparation

Choose a spacious and safe area where you can move freely without constraints.

Wear comfortable clothing that doesn't restrict your movements.

Set aside time for both free-form and structured activities without rushing.

### Tips & Advice

In free-form movement, let go of any judgments or expectations. Allow your body to express itself freely.

In structured movement, respect your body's limits and focus on precision and control.

Use music if it helps you engage more deeply in the movement.

### Step-by-Step Instructions

**Free-form Movement:**

1. Begin by standing in an open space. Close your eyes and take a few deep breaths to center yourself.

2. Start moving your body in any way that feels natural. There's no right or wrong way to do this. Let your body lead the movement, not your mind.

3. Allow yourself to sway, stretch, bend, twist, or even dance. Focus on how each movement feels in your body.

4. Continue for as long as you feel comfortable, exploring different ranges and types of movement.

**Structured Movement:**

1. Choose a set of structured movements or poses, such as yoga, Tai Chi, or a simple stretching routine. You can also follow a guided video if preferred.

2. Perform each movement with mindfulness, paying attention to the alignment of your body, the sensations in each position, and the rhythm of your breathing.

3. Transition smoothly from one movement to the next, maintaining a focus on your body's responses.

**Reflection and Integration:**

1. After completing both free-form and structured movements, sit or lie down in a comfortable position.

2. Reflect on the experiences of both types of movement. How did your body feel during free-form movement compared to structured movement?

3. Consider the emotional and mental effects of each practice. Did one feel more relaxed or energized than the other?

## EMOTIONAL AWARENESS JOURNALING

This practice encourages mindfulness about your feelings and their physical manifestations in your body. It's about observing, acknowledging, and expressing your emotions in a safe, reflective space.

Aim to engage in Emotional Awareness Journaling daily, especially during times of emotional upheaval or stress. Even a few minutes can be beneficial.

### Objectives

To develop a deeper awareness of your emotional experiences.

To explore the connection between emotions and bodily sensations.

To cultivate a habit of self-reflection and emotional expression

### Preparation

Choose a quiet and comfortable space for journaling where you won't be interrupted.

Have a journal or notebook dedicated to this practice, along with a pen or pencil.

Set aside a regular time each day for this practice, if possible.

### Tips & Advice

Be as honest and open as possible with your feelings.

Don't worry about grammar or spelling; focus on expressing yourself freely.

Consider using prompts if you're unsure where to start, such as "Right now, I feel...", "Today, I noticed...", or "I am surprised by...".

### Step-by-Step Instructions

**Setting the Stage:**

1. Begin with a few deep, calming breaths to center yourself.

2. If helpful, do a brief body scan to become present in the moment.

**Journaling Process:**

1. Start by writing down how you are feeling at this moment. Don't censor or judge your feelings; simply acknowledge them as they are.

2. Reflect on where in your body you might be experiencing these emotions. Describe any physical sensations, like tightness in the chest, a knot in the stomach, or a sense of warmth.

**Exploring Emotions:**

1. If a particular emotion is prominent, explore it further. Ask yourself: What might be triggering this emotion? Have I felt this way before? What thoughts are associated with this feeling?

2. Remember, there are no right or wrong answers. This is a process of exploration and self-discovery.

**Reflecting on Patterns:**

1. Notice if there are any recurring emotions or bodily sensations that appear in your journal over time. Are there patterns related to specific times, events, or interactions?

2. Reflect on how acknowledging these emotions and feel. Do you notice any shifts in your emotional state after journaling?

**Closing the Session:**

1. Conclude your journaling session with a few calming breaths.

2. Express gratitude to yourself for taking the time to connect with your emotions and body.

# GROUNDING TECHNIQUES

Grounding techniques are essential in somatic therapy for establishing a sense of presence and stability, especially in moments of stress or disconnection. These techniques help bring your awareness back to the present moment and to your physical body, anchoring you in the 'here and now.' They also have the power of reducing symptoms of anxiety, dissociation, or emotional distress and therefore, they help cultivate a sense of physical and emotional stability.

Experiment with different grounding techniques to find what works best for you.

Grounding can be practiced multiple times a day, especially in moments of anxiety or disconnection.

After practicing a grounding technique, take a moment to notice any changes in your body or mind.

## Most Effective Technique

**Reflect on which technique is the most effective for you and decide how you might integrate it into your daily routine.**

## FIVE SENSES GROUNDING:

1. Take a deep breath and slowly exhale.
2. Name 5 things you can see around you.
3. Identify 4 things you can touch or feel (the texture of your clothes, the ground under your feet).
4. Listen for 3 things you can hear in the immediate environment.
5. Notice 2 things you can smell or, if that's not applicable, two smells you like.
6. Think of 1 thing you can taste or like the taste of.

## VISUALIZATION FOR GROUNDING:

1. Close your eyes and imagine roots growing from the soles of your feet into the ground.
2. Visualize these roots anchoring you firmly to the earth.
3. With each breath, imagine drawing strength and stability from the ground into your body.

## GROUNDING THROUGH BREATH:

1. Sit comfortably with your feet flat on the ground.
2. Take slow, deep breaths. Inhale through your nose, counting to four, hold for a count of four, then exhale through your mouth for a count of six.
3. As you breathe, focus on the sensation of air entering and leaving your body, and your feet's connection to the ground.

## PHYSICAL GROUNDING WITH OBJECTS:

1. Hold a small object (like a stone, a small ball, or a textured fabric) in your hand.
2. Focus on the texture, temperature, and weight of the object.
3. If your mind wanders, gently bring your attention back to the sensations in your hand.

## MOVEMENT-BASED GROUNDING:

1. Stand up and gently sway from side to side or march in place.
2. Pay attention to the sensations in your legs and feet as they move and touch the ground.
3. Use this movement to reconnect with your body and the present moment.

## EXERCISE TO CONNECT WITH THE PRESENT MOMENT

Connecting with the present moment is designed to help you cultivate a deeper sense of awareness and presence, reducing feelings of stress and anxiety by focusing on the 'now.'

### Objectives

To enhance present-moment awareness.

To reduce the impact of distracting thoughts and worries about the past or future.

To cultivate a sense of calm and focus.

### Preparation

Choose a quiet place where you can sit or stand comfortably without interruptions.

Find a comfortable position. If seated, ensure your feet are flat on the ground. If standing, stand firmly and balanced.

Allocate a few minutes where you can practice without hurry.

### Tips & Advice

Practice this exercise regularly to become more adept at bringing yourself back to the present moment.

If your mind wanders, gently guide it back without judgment.

Modify the exercise to suit your needs and preferences, focusing more on the senses that most effectively help you ground in the present.

### Step-by-Step Instructions

**Engaging the Senses:**

1. Close your eyes gently and take a few deep breaths. As you breathe in and out, allow your body to relax.
2. Open your eyes and focus on your surroundings. Identify and acknowledge five things you can see. Take a moment to really look at them and notice their details – color, texture, shape.
3. Now, focus on four things you can touch. It can be the chair you are sitting on, the ground under your feet, the air against your skin, or your clothes against your body. Notice the textures and temperatures.
4. Concentrate on three things you can hear. These might be distant sounds or those close by. Listen to the quality and layers of these sounds.
5. Identify two things you can smell. If you can't immediately smell anything, recall two of your favorite scents.
6. Focus on one thing you can taste. It might be the lingering taste of a meal, a drink, or just the sensation of your mouth.

**Connecting with Your Breath:**

1. Return your focus to your breathing. Breathe slowly and deeply, feeling each breath as it moves in and out of your body.
2. With each exhale, imagine releasing any tension or stress. With each inhale, think of drawing in peace and calm.

**Body Awareness:**

1. Pay attention to your body. Notice any sensations, tension, or relaxation in different areas. Don't judge or try to change these sensations, just observe them.

**Acknowledging Thoughts:**

1. As thoughts come into your mind, acknowledge them and then gently let them go. Imagine them as clouds passing in the sky, neither clinging to them nor pushing them away.

**Concluding the Exercise:**

1. Take a few more deep breaths and then slowly bring your awareness back to the room.

## Journaling and Integration

After completing the exercise, reflect on your experience. Did you find certain senses more dominant? How do you feel now compared to before the exercise? Consider how you can use this technique in daily life, perhaps in moments of stress or when you need to refocus.

## BODY INTUITION

Developing body intuition involves learning how to tune into and interpret the signals your body sends. This practice enhances your ability to understand and respond to your body's needs, leading to greater self-awareness and well-being.

This practice can be done daily or as often as you find helpful. Regular practice will enhance your ability to intuitively understand and respond to your body's signals.

### Objectives

To increase awareness of bodily sensations and signals.

To cultivate a deeper connection and understanding of your body.

To improve decision-making regarding health, comfort, and emotional needs.

### Preparation

Find a quiet, comfortable space where you can relax without interruption.

Wear clothing that is comfortable and allows you to feel unrestricted.

Allocate time when you can focus without feeling rushed.

### Tips & Advice

Practice this exercise regularly to become more attuned to your body's signals.

Be open and curious about what your body is communicating, without preconceived notions.

Use your findings to make informed decisions about self-care, exercise, rest, and other needs.

### Step-by-Step Instructions

**Relaxation and Centering:**

1. Begin by sitting or lying in a comfortable position. Close your eyes and take several deep, slow breaths.

2. Allow your body to relax with each exhale. Try to release tension from your muscles and clear your mind of distractions.

**Body Scan for Awareness:**

1. Slowly guide your attention through your body, starting from the toes and moving upwards.

2. Notice any sensations in each part of the body – tension, relaxation, warmth, coolness, tingling, or numbness.

3. Try not to judge or change these sensations, just observe them as they are.

**Identifying Bodily Signals:**

1. Pay attention to areas in your body that might be communicating discomfort, pain, or ease.

2. Acknowledge any emotional sensations that arise with these physical feelings. For instance, do certain areas of tension correlate with feelings of stress or anxiety?

**Reflecting on Responses:**

1. Consider how your body reacts to different situations, emotions, or environments. Do certain scenarios cause physical discomfort or relaxation?

2. Reflect on how your body communicates hunger, fatigue, or the need for movement, stillness, or elimination.

After completing the body scan, take some time to journal about your experience. Note any patterns or discoveries you made about your bodily signals. This can help in recognizing and responding to these signals more effectively in the future.

# PROGRESS TRACKING CHART

As you embark on this transformative journey with your workbook, I introduce an essential component right from the start: the Progress Tracking section. This feature is a core part of your journey, designed to accompany you from the very beginning. This section is a space where you can chart the evolution of your experiences, emotions, and discoveries as you navigate through each exercise. It stands as a proactive tool for reflection, allowing you to document your journey, celebrate your progress, and ponder over the areas ripe for deeper exploration. By integrating this tracking at the outset, the importance of mindfulness and self reflection is emphasized in your personal growth. It encourages you to engage actively with your transformation, fostering a deeper connection with your inner self. This practice not only offers you clarity and insight into your patterns and challenges but also celebrates your achievements and the subtle yet significant shifts in your journey.

Approach this section—and indeed, the entire workbook—with openness, curiosity, and compassion for yourself. Let it guide you, inspire you, and remind you of your commitment to self-exploration and healing. Your journey through this workbook is unique to you, and the Progress Tracking section is here to ensure you recognize and honor every step on your path to greater self-awareness and well-being.

**Date:**

| Exercise | Duration (Minutes) | Emotional State Before | Emotional State After | Physical Sensations | Insights Gained | Areas for Improvement |
|---|---|---|---|---|---|---|
|  |  |  |  |  |  |  |

**Date:**

| Exercise | Duration (Minutes) | Emotional State Before | Emotional State After | Physical Sensations | Insights Gained | Areas for Improvement |
|---|---|---|---|---|---|---|
|  |  |  |  |  |  |  |

**Date:**

| Exercise | Duration (Minutes) | Emotional State Before | Emotional State After | Physical Sensations | Insights Gained | Areas for Improvement |
|---|---|---|---|---|---|---|
|  |  |  |  |  |  |  |

**Date:**

| Exercise | Duration (Minutes) | Emotional State Before | Emotional State After | Physical Sensations | Insights Gained | Areas for Improvement |
|---|---|---|---|---|---|---|
|  |  |  |  |  |  |  |

**Date:**

| Exercise | Duration (Minutes) | Emotional State Before | Emotional State After | Physical Sensations | Insights Gained | Areas for Improvement |
|---|---|---|---|---|---|---|
|  |  |  |  |  |  |  |

**Date:**

| Exercise | Duration (Minutes) | Emotional State Before | Emotional State After | Physical Sensations | Insights Gained | Areas for Improvement |
|---|---|---|---|---|---|---|
|  |  |  |  |  |  |  |

**Date:**

| Exercise | Duration (Minutes) | Emotional State Before | Emotional State After | Physical Sensations | Insights Gained | Areas for Improvement |
|---|---|---|---|---|---|---|
|  |  |  |  |  |  |  |

**Date:**

| Exercise | Duration (Minutes) | Emotional State Before | Emotional State After | Physical Sensations | Insights Gained | Areas for Improvement |
|---|---|---|---|---|---|---|
|  |  |  |  |  |  |  |

| Date: | | | | | | |
|---|---|---|---|---|---|---|
| Exercise | Duration (Minutes) | Emotional State Before | Emotional State After | Physical Sensations | Insights Gained | Areas for Improvement |
| | | | | | | |

| Date: | | | | | | |
|---|---|---|---|---|---|---|
| Exercise | Duration (Minutes) | Emotional State Before | Emotional State After | Physical Sensations | Insights Gained | Areas for Improvement |
| | | | | | | |

| Date: | | | | | | |
|---|---|---|---|---|---|---|
| Exercise | Duration (Minutes) | Emotional State Before | Emotional State After | Physical Sensations | Insights Gained | Areas for Improvement |
| | | | | | | |

| Date: | | | | | | |
|---|---|---|---|---|---|---|
| Exercise | Duration (Minutes) | Emotional State Before | Emotional State After | Physical Sensations | Insights Gained | Areas for Improvement |
| | | | | | | |

| Date: | | | | | | |
|---|---|---|---|---|---|---|
| Exercise | Duration (Minutes) | Emotional State Before | Emotional State After | Physical Sensations | Insights Gained | Areas for Improvement |
| | | | | | | |

**Date:**

| Exercise | Duration (Minutes) | Emotional State Before | Emotional State After | Physical Sensations | Insights Gained | Areas for Improvement |
|---|---|---|---|---|---|---|
| | | | | | | |

**Date:**

| Exercise | Duration (Minutes) | Emotional State Before | Emotional State After | Physical Sensations | Insights Gained | Areas for Improvement |
|---|---|---|---|---|---|---|
| | | | | | | |

**Date:**

| Exercise | Duration (Minutes) | Emotional State Before | Emotional State After | Physical Sensations | Insights Gained | Areas for Improvement |
|---|---|---|---|---|---|---|
| | | | | | | |

**Date:**

| Exercise | Duration (Minutes) | Emotional State Before | Emotional State After | Physical Sensations | Insights Gained | Areas for Improvement |
|---|---|---|---|---|---|---|
| | | | | | | |

**Date:**

| Exercise | Duration (Minutes) | Emotional State Before | Emotional State After | Physical Sensations | Insights Gained | Areas for Improvement |
|---|---|---|---|---|---|---|
| | | | | | | |

# WORKING THROUGHT TRAUMA

## SAFE SPACE CREATION: ESTABLISHING BOUNDARIES AND SAFETY IN PRACTICE

Creating a safe space, both physically and emotionally, is crucial when engaging in somatic practices, especially when working through trauma. This means creating and ensuring a sense of safety that allows you to be vulnerable; engage in this practice as often as needed, especially before beginning any work related to trauma processing or deep emotional exploration.

## Objectives

To create an environment that feels secure and supportive for trauma work.

To establish boundaries that respect personal comfort and limits.

To cultivate a sense of safety that facilitates healing and exploration.

## Preparation

Choose a quiet, private space where you can be undisturbed.

Ensure the space is comfortable and soothing. This might include comfortable seating, soft lighting, and a temperature that feels right.

Have any supportive items on hand, such as blankets, cushions, or objects that provide comfort.

## Tips & Advice

Respect your own needs and adjust the space and practice as needed.

Regularly reassess your boundaries and safety needs as they might change over time.

Remember that creating a safe space is an ongoing process, not a one-time setup.

## Step-by-Step Instructions

### Physical Space Preparation:

1. Arrange the physical space to promote relaxation and security. This might mean adjusting lighting, clearing clutter, or setting up a comfortable place to sit or lie down.

2. Consider the use of calming elements like soft music, gentle scents, or soothing colors.

### Mental and Emotional Preparation:

1. Before beginning any trauma-related work, take time to mentally prepare. This might involve deep breathing, a short meditation, or setting intentions for the session.

2. Remind yourself that you are in a safe space and have control over the session. You can pause, modify, or stop the practice at any time.

### Establishing Boundaries:

1. Reflect on and establish your personal boundaries. Determine what you are and aren't comfortable with in your practice.

### Creating an Emotional Safety Net:

1. Have a plan for managing intense emotions or physical responses that might arise. This could include breathing techniques, taking a break, or having a support person to contact.

2. Keep a journal or other means of expression nearby to document your experiences and feelings as needed.

### Concluding the Session:

1. At the end of your practice, take time to decompress and gently transition back to your usual activities.

2. Engage in a soothing activity that helps ground you, like walking, drinking tea, or listening to music.

# My Boundaries

Consider your personal boundaries in relation to healing and self-care. Ask yourself these guiding questions: What activities or environments comfort or disturb you? What do you need to feel safe and supported during your practice? Reflect on these points to understand your boundaries better.

# My Emotional Safety Nest

Think about what makes a space feel safe and soothing to you. Consider aspects like lighting, scents, textures, or colors. What objects or keepsakes bring comfort or positive memories? What rituals or activities could enhance your sense of safety and peace?

## EXERCISE FOR RELEASING TRAUMATIC ENERGY STORED IN THE BODY

Trauma can often manifest as stored energy in the body, leading to physical tension and emotional distress. This exercise is designed to help release that energy in a safe and controlled manner, aiding in the healing process. Practice this exercise as needed, especially when feeling physically tense or emotionally burdened; regular practice can aid in managing and processing trauma-related stress.

 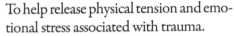

### Objectives

To help release physical tension and emotional stress associated with trauma.

To promote relaxation and restoration of balance in the body and mind.

To facilitate a sense of release and relief from trauma-related symptoms

### Preparation

Find a private, comfortable space where you feel secure and won't be disturbed.

Wear comfortable clothing that allows for unrestricted movement.

Have a supportive surface such as a yoga mat or soft rug.

### Tips & Advice

Listen to your body and respect its limits. Do not force any movement that feels uncomfortable or painful.

Be patient with the process, as releasing stored trauma can take time and may need to be revisited.

It's normal for emotions to surface during this exercise. Allow yourself to experience and express these emotions safely.

### Step-by-Step Instructions

1. **Grounding and Centering:**

Begin by grounding yourself in the present moment. Sit or stand in a comfortable position, take deep breaths, and focus on your connection to the ground beneath you.

2. **Recognizing Body Tension:**

Perform a gentle body scan to identify areas where you feel tension or discomfort. Acknowledge these areas without judgment.

3. **Engaging in Mindful Movement:**

Start with gentle movements, such as stretching or swaying. Pay attention to how your body feels and respond to its needs. Gradually increase the intensity if it feels right. This could include shaking your limbs, dancing freely, or doing more vigorous stretches.

4. **Breathwork for Release:**

Incorporate deep, controlled breathing. Inhale deeply, then exhale forcefully, imagining the release of traumatic energy with each breath. You might vocalize on the exhale, such as sighing or making a sound, to enhance the sense of release.

5. **Soothing and Calming the Body:**

After the active release, gradually slow your movements. Transition into more calming activities, such as gentle yoga poses, slow walking, or rocking your body.

6. **Concluding with Reflection:**

Once you feel your energy has shifted and you are ready to conclude, sit down comfortably. Reflect on the experience and any sensations or emotions that arose. Journaling about the experience can be helpful.

# CONNECTION BETWEEN EMOTIONS AND THEIR PHYSICAL MANIFESTATIONS

## Chest

The chest, particularly the heart area, is often associated with emotions related to love, joy, heartache, and grief.

When experiencing love or joy, you might feel a sense of warmth or expansion in the chest.

Conversely, during heartache or grief, there may be sensations of tightness, heaviness, or aching in this area.

Tuning into these sensations can provide clues about your emotional state and needs related to connection and loss.

## Stomach

The stomach or abdominal area is commonly linked to emotions like fear, anxiety, and nervousness.

Physical sensations might include "butterflies," a churning feeling, or a sense of tightness or knots in the stomach.

These sensations are often part of the body's natural response to perceived threats or stressors and can be cues to engage in practices that promote safety.

## Throat

The throat can reflect emotions related to sadness, grief, or the need to express thoughts and feelings.

A lump in the throat or a tight feeling may be experienced during intense sadness or when you feel the need to cry but are holding back tears.

Feelings of constriction or pressure in the throat could also signify the need to communicate or express something that has been left unsaid or suppressed.

## Forehead and Eyes

Tension or pain in the forehead and around the eyes can be associated with stress, worry, or deep concentration.

A furrowed brow or a headache, especially around the temples, can indicate mental strain or overthinking.

Relaxation techniques focusing on the head area can help in alleviating these symptoms and bring awareness to the need for mental rest or clarity.

## Legs

Legs, particularly the thighs, can hold tension related to forward movement in life, including fears or hesitations about the future.

Weakness or instability in the legs might reflect a lack of grounding or uncertainty in one's life path.

Strong, stable legs can indicate a sense of confidence and progress, suggesting a feeling of being well-grounded and secure in one's journey.

## Knees

The knees can symbolize flexibility and vulnerability. Issues with the knees might indicate difficulty in bending or yielding in situations, symbolizing stubbornness or ego issues.

Pain or discomfort in the knees can also point to a deep-seated fear of vulnerability or an unwillingness to be flexible in thoughts or actions.

## Feet

The feet are our primary connection to the earth and can represent our foundation and sense of stability.

Problems with the feet, such as pain or discomfort, might suggest issues with moving forward in life, feeling "stuck," or difficulty in finding one's footing in new situations.

Taking care of the feet, through grounding exercises or mindful walking, can enhance a sense of connection with the earth and a feeling of being supported in life's journey.

## Lower Back

Lower back discomfort can be linked to feelings of insecurity, financial stress, or lack of emotional support.

Chronic lower back pain might indicate deep-seated fears or unresolved emotional issues relating to stability and support in life.

## Ankles

The ankles offer support and flexibility in movement and can reflect our ability to receive pleasure and joy in life.

Stiffness or pain in the ankles might indicate resistance to allowing oneself to experience joy or a lack of flexibility in adapting to life's changes.

Healthy, flexible ankles can symbolize the ease of moving through life's ups and downs and the ability to navigate changes with grace.

## Shoulders and Upper Back

The shoulders and upper back often bear physical tension related to stress, responsibility, or burdens.

A feeling of weight or tightness in these areas might suggest carrying emotional weight or a feeling of being overwhelmed.

Mindful movement and awareness practices can help in releasing this tension and exploring the underlying emotions.

## Hands and Arms

Emotions like anger, frustration, or a desire to control situations can manifest as tension or clenching in the hands and arms.

Conversely, open and relaxed hands and arms may indicate feelings of openness, acceptance, and readiness to connect with others.

## Hips

The hips are often considered a storage area for emotions, particularly those related to control, fear, and trauma.

Tightness or stiffness in the hips can be a physical manifestation of resistance to change or holding onto past experiences and emotions.

Opening and releasing tension in the hip area through stretches or movement can sometimes lead to the release of emotional blockages and increased flexibility, both physically and emotionally.

# IDENTIFYING AND EXPRESSING EMOTIONS THROUGH THE BODY

This exercise is about recognizing and expressing emotions through bodily sensations. Often, emotions are stored and experienced in the body, and learning to identify and express them can be a powerful tool for emotional regulation and self-awareness. Practice this exercise when you feel emotionally overwhelmed or disconnected from your feelings.

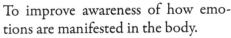

## Objectives

To improve awareness of how emotions are manifested in the body.

Learn how to express and manage emotions through bodily awareness.

To use the body as a tool for emotional release and processing.

## Preparation

Find a private, comfortable space where you feel secure and won't be disturbed.

Wear comfortable clothing that allows for unrestricted movement.

Have a supportive surface such as a yoga mat or soft rug.

## Tips & Advice

Be patient and open to whatever arises. Some emotions may be more difficult to access or express than others.

Remember that movement and bodily expression do not need to be graceful or structured; it's about what feels right for you.

If strong emotions arise, remind yourself that this is a normal part of the healing process and stay present with your experience.

## Step-by-Step Instructions

### Body Scan for Emotional Awareness:

1. Begin by sitting or lying in a comfortable position. Close your eyes and take deep, slow breaths to center yourself.
2. Perform a body scan, starting from your toes and moving upwards, paying attention to any sensations or emotions in various parts of your body.
3. Notice areas of tension, relaxation, warmth, coolness, or tingling, and consider what emotions these sensations might be connected to.

### Connecting Emotions with Physical Sensations:

1. Focus on areas of the body where emotions seem most present. Common areas include the chest (for love and heartache), stomach (for fear and anxiety), and throat (for sadness or the need to express something).
2. Identify the emotion and explore it. Ask yourself: What is this feeling? Why might it be here? What does it need?

### Expressing Emotions Through Movement:

1. Allow your body to express the identified emotion through movement. This could be through dance, stretching, shaking, or any other movement that feels natural.
2. Focus on how the movement changes the sensations in your body and whether it alters the intensity of the emotion.

### Using Breath to Process Emotions:

1. Incorporate deep, conscious breathing. Imagine breathing into the areas where emotions are stored and visualize exhaling the emotion, releasing it from your body.
2. You may vocalize on the exhale to enhance the sense of release.

# Journaling and Reflection

After the exercise, take some time to journal about your experience. What did you notice about your emotional and physical state? Reflect on how identifying and expressing your emotions through the body felt different from just thinking about them.

## JOURNAL PROMPTS FOR PROCESSING TRAUMATIC EXPERIENCES

### Describing the Experience

"Describe the traumatic event or experience as if you were telling it to a stranger.
What details stand out the most?"

## JOURNAL PROMPTS FOR PROCESSING TRAUMATIC EXPERIENCES

**Emotional Response**

"What emotions did you feel during and immediately after the traumatic experience? Have these emotions changed over time?"

## JOURNAL PROMPTS FOR PROCESSING TRAUMATIC EXPERIENCES

### Physical Sensations

"Did you notice any physical reactions or sensations in your body during or after the traumatic experience? How does your body react when you think about it now?"

## JOURNAL PROMPTS FOR PROCESSING TRAUMATIC EXPERIENCES

### Thought Patterns

"What thoughts or beliefs about yourself, others, or the world have emerged since this traumatic event?"

## JOURNAL PROMPTS FOR PROCESSING TRAUMATIC EXPERIENCES

### Coping Mechanisms

"What coping strategies have you used to deal with trauma? Which have been helpful, and which have not?"

## JOURNAL PROMPTS FOR PROCESSING TRAUMATIC EXPERIENCES

### Personal Strengths

"Reflect on the strengths and resources you have used to survive and cope. What are they, and how have they helped you?"

## JOURNAL PROMPTS FOR PROCESSING TRAUMATIC EXPERIENCES

### Lessons and Insights

"Are there any lessons, insights, or new understandings you've gained about yourself or life as a result of this traumatic experience?"

## JOURNAL PROMPTS FOR PROCESSING TRAUMATIC EXPERIENCES

**Healing and Moving Forward**

"What does healing from this trauma look like for you? What steps can you take to move towards healing?"

## JOURNAL PROMPTS FOR PROCESSING TRAUMATIC EXPERIENCES

### Messages to Self

"Write a letter to yourself during the time of the trauma. What do you want to tell your past self?"

## JOURNAL PROMPTS FOR PROCESSING TRAUMATIC EXPERIENCES

### Imagining a Future

"Visualize where you want to be in terms of healing and personal growth. What does this look like, and what changes do you hope to see, feel, experince?"

# HOLISTIC TENSION RELEASE

## DYNAMIC TENSION AND RELEASE

Dynamic Tension and Release is an engaging exercise designed to heighten bodily awareness and facilitate emotional relief by actively engaging muscles in tension and then consciously releasing them. This practice not only aids in releasing physical tension but also helps in discharging emotional stress, creating a profound sense of relaxation and well-being. Overall, it is an effective addition to any routine focused on stress management, emotional, physical and mental regulation. This exercise can be practiced daily or as needed, especially during times of heightened stress or when you notice significant tension buildup in your body.

## Objectives

To identify and release stored tension in the body through controlled tension and relaxation of muscle groups.

To enhance mind-body connection by consciously engaging with and releasing physical tension.

To utilize the physical act of release as a metaphor for letting go of emotional and mental stress.

## Preparation

Choose a quiet, comfortable space where you can move freely and lie down.

Prepare to engage all major muscle groups, from your feet to your facial muscles.

## Tips & Advice

Pay particular attention to areas where you commonly hold stress and spend extra time working through these muscle groups.

Practice mindfulness during the exercise by focusing intently on the sensations of tension and release, using this as a method to stay present.

Consider using this exercise as a tool for managing stress and anxiety, recognizing the power of physical release in facilitating emotional relief.

## Step-by-Step Instructions

### Beginning with Grounding:

1. Start in a comfortable standing or sitting position, taking a few deep breaths to center yourself.

2. Close your eyes if comfortable, and bring your attention to your body, noticing any areas of tension.

### Engaging Muscle Groups:

1. Begin with your feet. Tense the muscles as tightly as possible for 5-10 seconds, then release suddenly and notice the sensation of relaxation.

2. Progressively move up the body, engaging and releasing each muscle group in turn: calves, thighs, buttocks, abdomen, chest, arms, hands, neck, and face.

### Focusing on Breath:

1. Coordinate your breathing with the exercise by inhaling deeply as you tense your muscles and exhaling forcefully as you release them.

2. Use your breath as a vehicle to enhance the sensation of tension release throughout your body.

### Observing and Reflecting:

1. After completing the muscle groups, lie down or sit comfortably. Take a moment to scan your body, observing any changes in physical sensation or emotional state.

**Reflect on the experience. How did actively engaging with tension and consciously releasing it affect your sense of well-being?**

## HOLISTIC TENSION RELEASE

## BREATHING EXERCISE FOR PAIN RELIEF

This exercise focuses on utilizing deep, mindful breathing to soothe the nervous system, reduce the intensity of pain perception, and promote relaxation of both the mind and body. By consciously altering our breathing patterns, we can tap into the body's natural ability to ease phycological, emotional and physical discomfort. Practice daily or whenever pain arises. Consistency can lead to better pain management and overall comfort.

### Objectives

To engage the body's natural pain relief system by activating the parasympathetic nervous system.

To distract from and lessen the perception of pain.

### Preparation

Find a quiet, comfortable space where you can sit or recline without interruptions.

Use cushions or props to support any painful areas and to ensure maximum comfort.

Choose a duration that feels manageable, starting with shorter sessions and gradually increasing as needed.

### Tips & Advice

Use visualization alongside breathing to enhance the pain-relief effect.

Practice consistently, as regular breathing exercises can increase your body's ability to manage pain.

Remain patient and gentle with yourself, acknowledging that pain management is a process.

### Step-by-Step Instructions

**Finding a Comfortable Rhythm:**

1. Begin by observing your natural breath without trying to change it.
2. Gradually start to deepen your inhales and lengthen your exhales, establishing a soothing rhythm.

**Engaging Diaphragmatic Breathing:**

1. Place one hand on your chest and the other on your belly. Breathe in such a way that only the hand on your belly rises.
2. Imagine your breath reaching the areas of pain, bringing warmth and relaxation to those parts with each inhalation.

**Synchronizing Breath with Movement:**

1. If comfortable, incorporate gentle movement, such as slowly rocking your feet or hands, synchronized with your breathing.
2. With each exhale, visualize the pain diminishing, like a wave receding from the shore.

**Progressive Muscle Relaxation:**

1. Tense each muscle group as you breathe in, and relax them as you breathe out, starting from your toes and moving up to your head.
2. Pay particular attention to the areas where you feel pain, directing your breath to release tension there.

**Closing the Practice:**

1. After completing your breathing cycles, take a moment to rest in the natural rhythm of your breath, noticing any changes in your pain levels.
2. Gently wiggle your fingers and toes, and when ready, open your eyes, returning to your day with a renewed sense of calm.

## Reflection

Reflect on the effect the breathing exercise had on your pain levels.

## Application

Consider how you can incorporate these breathing techniques during moments of discomfort that might occur throughout your day.

# VOCAL TONING AND HUMMING

Vocal Toning and Humming is a soothing exercise that uses the sound and vibration of your own voice to relax and release tension within the body. It's an effective way to engage the body and mind, utilizing the therapeutic power of sound to enhance well-being. Incorporate this exercise into your daily routine, especially during times of stress or when you feel the need for emotional grounding.

## Objectives

To utilize vocal sounds to create internal vibrations that massage and release muscular tension.

To promote relaxation and reduce stress through mindful sound production.

To connect with and regulate emotional states through tonal frequencies.

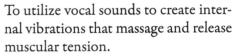

## Preparation

Find a quiet and comfortable space where you feel free to vocalize without inhibition.

Sit or stand in a relaxed posture, ensuring you're not constricted in any way.

Take a few deep breaths to center yourself and relax your body.

## Tips & Advice

Stay hydrated to keep your vocal cords lubricated.

Be mindful of not straining your voice; the goal is gentle vibration and relaxation.

Practice regularly to deepen the connection between sound, body, and emotion.

## Step-by-Step Instructions

### Beginning with Humming:

1. Start by gently closing your lips and taking a deep breath through your nose.

2. On the exhale, produce a humming sound, feeling the vibration primarily in your head and chest.

3. Experiment with different pitches to find the tone that feels most soothing.

### Progressing to Toning:

1. Open your mouth slightly and transition from humming to toning, using vowel sounds such as "ah," "oh," or "ee."

2. Focus on the sensation of vibration in different parts of your body. Notice how changing pitches affects where you feel the vibration.

3. Allow the sound to resonate freely, paying attention to the release of tension.

### Exploring Emotional Release:

1. Identify any areas of emotional tension in your body and direct your tone to these areas. Imagine the sound vibrating and loosening the emotional knots.

2. Notice any emotions that arise as you tone. Allow these feelings to be expressed and released through your voice.

### Concluding with Silence:

1. After toning, rest in silence for a few minutes. Observe the sensations in your body and the state of your mind.

2. Reflect on the experience of using your voice as a tool for inner massage and emotional release.

## Journaling and Reflection

How did the integration of mind, body, and emotional practices affect your experience of tension and pain? Were there any moments of unexpected insight or relief? Note any shifts in your physical sensations, emotional states, or thoughts before and after the exercises.

## CONCENTRATION MEDITATION

Concentration Meditation is a practice that hones your ability to focus on a single point of reference. This focused approach can help anchor the mind, bringing heightened awareness to physical sensations. By fostering this state of concentration, you become more attuned to your body, allowing for greater identification, processing, and release of stored tensions. This practice not only sharpens the mind but also paves the way for a more introspective and embodied healing process, where you can gently observe and address the somatic nuances of emotional experiences.

### Objectives

To sharpen mental focus and reduce the frequency of distracting thoughts.

To improve concentration and mental discipline.

To create a sense of inner calm that can enhance all areas of life.

### Preparation

Find a quiet space where you can sit undisturbed and ensure comfortable seating.

Choose an object of focus, such as a candle flame, or a simple, repetitive sound like a metronome or a bell.

Decide the duration of your meditation session. Start with a few minutes and gradually increase as your concentration improves.

### Tips & Advice

Keep the sessions short initially to avoid frustration and gradually increase the time as your concentration builds.

Practice at the same time each day to develop a consistent routine.

Ensure that your object or sound of focus is not overly stimulating or complex, as the goal is to calm and collect the mind.

### Step-by-Step Instructions

**Settling In:**

1. Sit comfortably with a straight yet relaxed posture. Rest your hands on your lap or knees.

2. Take a few deep breaths to relax your body and signal the transition into a meditative state.

**Engaging with Your Focus Point:**

1. Gently rest your gaze on the candle flame or close your eyes if focusing on a sound.

2. Allow all other thoughts to fade into the background as you bring your full attention to the object or sound.

**Maintaining Focus:**

1. If your mind wanders, acknowledge the distraction and then gently redirect your focus back to the chosen object or sound.

2. With each moment of focus, deepen your state of concentration, letting go of external concerns.

**Deepening the Practice:**

1. As you become more absorbed, you may find that your awareness of the object or sound becomes more nuanced and profound.

2. Remain patient and persistent, recognizing that mastery of concentration takes time and practice.

**Concluding Your Session:**

1. Before ending your meditation, take a moment to appreciate the stillness and focus you've cultivated.

2. Slowly expand your awareness back to your surroundings and carry the calmness with you as you resume your day.

## Journaling and Reflection

After the session, reflect on the quality of your concentration and the feelings it elicited. Did you find moments of true focus? Consider how this practice of single-pointed focus can be applied to daily tasks or activities that require concentration.

# MANAGING SYMPTOMS OF ANXIETY

## BREATHING PATTERNS ANALYSIS

Breathing Patterns Analysis is a reflective exercise aimed at understanding the intricate link between your breathing patterns and emotional states, particularly anxiety. By observing how your breath changes across different situations, you can learn to regulate your emotional responses more effectively. Aim to observe and record your breathing patterns at least twice a day for a period of one to two weeks. This regular practice will help you establish a baseline understanding of your natural breathing patterns and their impact on your emotional well-being.

### Objectives

Learn how different breathing patterns correlate with feelings of anxiety versus calmness.

To develop awareness of your natural breathing patterns during various emotional states.

To utilize breath control techniques to manage anxiety.

### Preparation

Find a quiet, comfortable space where you can observe your breathing without interruptions.

Choose times throughout the day when you can pause to monitor your breathing, including moments of both calmness and stress.

### Tips & Advice

Practice non-judgment as you observe your breathing patterns. This exercise is about awareness, not self-criticism.

Consistency in observation is key. Try to record your breathing patterns under various emotional states throughout the day for a comprehensive understanding.

Explore different breathing techniques to discover which are most effective for you in managing anxiety.

### Step-by-Step Instructions

**Baseline Breathing Observation:**

1. At a calm moment, sit or lie down in a comfortable position. Close your eyes and take a few deep breaths.

2. Observe your natural breathing pattern. Note the pace, depth, and whether your breath is more chest- or abdomen-focused.

**Anxiety Breathing Observation:**

1. During a moment of anxiety, pause to observe your breathing. Note any changes from your baseline observation.

2. Pay attention to whether your breathing becomes shallower, faster, or more chest-oriented.

**Recording Observations:**

1. In your journal or phone, record the characteristics of your breathing under both states. Include details about the depth, pace, and location of your breath.

2. Note any physical sensations or emotions that accompany each breathing pattern.

**Experimenting with Breath Control:**

1. When noticing anxious breathing patterns, consciously apply slow, deep abdominal breathing. Inhale deeply through your nose, allowing your abdomen to rise, and exhale slowly through your mouth.

2. Record any changes in your emotional state after applying these techniques.

## Baseline Breathing Observations - Week 1

| DAY | PEACE | DEPTH | FOCUS | PEACE | DEPTH | FOCUS |
|-----|-------|-------|-------|-------|-------|-------|
|     |       |       |       |       |       |       |
|     |       |       |       |       |       |       |
|     |       |       |       |       |       |       |
|     |       |       |       |       |       |       |
|     |       |       |       |       |       |       |
|     |       |       |       |       |       |       |
|     |       |       |       |       |       |       |

## Baseline Breathing Observations - Week 2

| DAY | PEACE | DEPTH | FOCUS | PEACE | DEPTH | FOCUS |
|-----|-------|-------|-------|-------|-------|-------|
|     |       |       |       |       |       |       |
|     |       |       |       |       |       |       |
|     |       |       |       |       |       |       |
|     |       |       |       |       |       |       |
|     |       |       |       |       |       |       |
|     |       |       |       |       |       |       |
|     |       |       |       |       |       |       |

# MANAGING SYMPTOMS OF ANXIETY

## VISUALIZATION TECHNIQUE FOR RELAXATION

Visualization involves using mental imagery to induce a state of relaxation and tranquility. By creating vivid, peaceful images in the mind, you can engage your body's natural relaxation response, which can help reduce stress and promote a sense of well-being. This visualization technique can be practiced as often as you like; Regular practice can help improve your ability to quickly enter a state of relaxation.

### Objectives

To calm the mind and reduce stress and anxiety.

To use the power of the imagination to induce physical relaxation.

To create a mental escape that fosters peace and serenity

### Preparation

Choose a quiet, comfortable place where you can sit or lie down without being disturbed.

Make sure you are in a comfortable position, and your environment is conducive to relaxation.

Decide on the duration of your practice, but even a short period of visualization can be beneficial.

### Tips & Advice

Choose imagery that is personally soothing and pleasant for you.

Don't worry if your images are not crystal clear; the intention is more important than perfect detail.

Practice regularly to enhance your ability to create vivid, relaxing imagery.

### Step-by-Step Instructions

1. **Getting into a Relaxed State:**

   1. Begin by taking several deep, slow breaths. With each exhale, allow any tension to leave your body.
   2. Close your eyes gently and continue to breathe slowly and deeply, creating a sense of calm throughout your body.

   **Creating Your Relaxing Scene:**

   1. In your mind, start to imagine a place where you feel completely at ease. This could be a real place you've visited before, or it can be completely imaginary.
   2. Picture the details of this place. What do you see around you? Are there any sounds, like the rustling of leaves, the sound of water, or the melody of birds? What do you feel? Is the sun warming your skin, or is there a gentle breeze? What scents are in the air?

   **Engaging the Senses:**

   1. Engage all your senses as you build this scene in your mind. The more detailed your visualization, the more immersive the experience.
   2. Imagine yourself moving through this space. What are you doing? How do you feel as you engage with this environment?

   **Deepening the Relaxation:**

   1. As you become more absorbed in your visualization, notice how your body responds. Feel yourself becoming more and more relaxed with each detail you add to your scene.
   2. If your mind starts to wander, gently bring it back to the imagery and sensations of your peaceful place.

   **Concluding the Visualization:**

   1. Spend a few more moments enjoying the serenity of your mental imagery.
   2. When you're ready, slowly start to bring your awareness back to the present. Wiggle your fingers and toes, take a deep breath, and open your eyes when you feel comfortable.

# MANAGING SYMPTOMS OF ANXIETY

## GROUNDING EXERCISE

Grounding exercises are techniques used to bring one's focus to the present moment, connecting to the physical sensations of the body and the immediate environment. This exercise can be done for a few minutes or longer, depending on your needs. It is suitable for frequent practice, especially during times of high stress or when you feel mentally scattered.

## Objectives

Helps in managing anxiety, panic attacks, and stress.

They are effective in bringing a sense of calm and focus, especially useful for those with PTSD, trauma, or heightened stress levels.

Anchoring oneself in times of emotional distress or disconnection.

## Preparation

Choose a comfortable seated, standing, or lying position in a quiet space where you can focus without interruption.

Decide on the duration of your practice, but even a short period of visualization can be beneficial.

## Tips & Advice

Practice deep, controlled breathing throughout these exercises to enhance the grounding effect.

For those who have difficulty with the five senses technique, focusing solely on breath or physical sensations (like touching a surface) can be an alternative.

Visual grounding can involve focusing on a photograph or a specific object.

If you become distracted, gently bring your attention back to the exercise without judgment.

## Step-by-Step Instructions

**Deep Breathing:**

1. Take slow, deep breaths. Inhale through your nose and exhale through your mouth.

2. Feel your chest and abdomen rise and fall.

**Physical Grounding:**

1. Press your feet firmly into the ground and notice the sensation of the Earth beneath you.

2. Clench your hands into fists, then release, noting the feeling of tension and relaxation.

**Five Senses Grounding Technique:**

1. Notice five things you can see around you and name them.

2. Acknowledge four things you can feel or touch (like the texture of your clothing or the air on your skin).

3. Listen for three sounds you can hear in your environment.

4. Identify two things you can smell. If you can't smell anything, think of your favorite scents.

5. Focus on one thing you can taste or remember a favorite taste.

**Reflection and Application:**

1. Conclude your grounding practice by slowly transitioning your focus back to your usual activities. Take a moment to appreciate the calm and centered state you have cultivated.

2. After practicing grounding exercises, reflect: "How do I feel now compared to before the exercise? What sensations or emotions did I notice during the practice?"

## JOURNAL PROMPTS FOR MANAGING SYMPTOMS OF ANXIETY

### Unpacking Anxiety's Message

"Consider a moment when anxiety was at its peak. What might this anxiety be trying to communicate to you about your needs, fears, or boundaries? Reflect on how acknowledging and addressing these underlying messages could alter your response to similar situations in the future?"

## JOURNAL PROMPTS FOR MANAGING SYMPTOMS OF ANXIETY

### Constructive Conversations with Anxiety

"If your anxiety could offer you constructive advice on how to alleviate its symptoms, what would it say? Reflect on this perspective and write a letter from your anxiety to you, detailing supportive steps you can take to manage its presence in your life more effectively."

## BODY SCAN MEDITATION

The Body Scan is a fundamental exercise in somatic therapy, designed to help you develop awareness of your body's sensations, both comfortable and uncomfortable. It's a form of mindfulness practice that encourages you to tune into your body and notice any areas of tension, relaxation, or neutrality. Practice this exercise daily or as often as you like. It can be particularly helpful during times of stress or when you need to reconnect with your body.

### Objectives

To identify and acknowledge physical sensations in different parts of your body.

To develop a deeper connection with your body.

To learn to observe bodily sensations without judgment.

### Preparation

Find a quiet, comfortable space where you won't be disturbed.

You can do this exercise lying down, sitting, or in any comfortable position.

Ensure you are warm enough, and your environment is conducive to relaxation.

### Tips & Advice

If your mind wanders, gently acknowledge it and return your focus to the body scan.

Approach each sensation with curiosity and without judgment.

Combine the body scan with deep breathing for enhanced relaxation. Each breath can help release tension and deepen your awareness.

Adjust your position if you become uncomfortable.

### Step-by-Step Instructions

**Beginning the Scan:**

1. Close your eyes gently and take a few deep breaths. Inhale slowly through your nose, hold for a moment, and exhale through your mouth. Allow your body to relax with each breath.

2. Start by bringing your attention to the top of your head. Notice any sensations here – it could be tightness, tingling, warmth, coolness, or nothing at all.

**Progressing Through the Body:**

1. Slowly move your attention down from the top of your head to your forehead, eyes, cheeks, and jaw. Spend a moment at each area, noticing any sensations or lack thereof.

2. Continue this process through each part of your body: neck, shoulders, arms, hands, chest, abdomen, back, hips, legs, and feet. Take your time to observe each area without rush.

**Observing Sensations:**

1. As you focus on each part of your body, observe any tension, pain, comfort, or other sensations. If you find areas of tension, acknowledge them without trying to change them.

2. If your mind wanders, gently bring your attention back to the part of the body you were focusing on.

**Completing the Scan:**

1. Once you reach your feet, take a few more deep breaths. Then, slowly wiggle your fingers and toes, bringing awareness back to your whole body.

2. Gently open your eyes. Take a moment to notice how your body feels as a whole. You might feel more relaxed or more attuned to sensations in your body.

# Journaling and Reflection

After completing the body scan, take a few minutes to reflect or journal about the experience. What did you notice? Were there areas of unexpected tension or relaxation? How do you feel emotionally after the scan?

# ENHANCING EMOTIONAL AWARENESS

## MIRROR WORK

Mirror work is a powerful practice aimed at improving self-esteem and fostering a positive relationship with oneself. This exercise involves direct engagement with your own reflection, using affirmations and compassionate dialogue to deepen self-understanding and acceptance. Daily practice is recommended, especially for beginners. Over time, you may adjust the frequency as you become more comfortable and attuned to the process.

### Objectives

To enhance self-love and acceptance through positive self-talk.

To confront and challenge negative beliefs about oneself.

To cultivate a nurturing and compassionate relationship with oneself.

### Preparation

Find a mirror in a private, comfortable space where you can speak to yourself without interruptions.

Choose a time of day when you feel most receptive and open—many find mornings ideal.

Have a list of affirmations or positive statements ready, or prepare to speak spontaneously from the heart.

### Tips & Advice

Mirror work can feel awkward or emotional at first. Be patient and kind with yourself as you navigate these feelings.

Tailor your affirmations to address your specific needs and challenges.

Consider keeping a journal to reflect on your experiences and progress with mirror work.

### Step-by-Step Instructions

**Engaging with Your Reflection:**

1. Stand or sit comfortably in front of the mirror. Look directly into your own eyes.

2. Take a few deep breaths to center yourself and create a sense of openness and receptivity.

**Speaking Affirmations:**

1. Begin by addressing yourself using your name or terms of endearment.

2. Slowly and clearly, speak your affirmations or positive statements. These could be phrases like "I am worthy of love and respect" or "I accept myself unconditionally."

3. Focus on the sincerity of your words, making an effort to truly feel their meaning.

**Reflecting on Your Thoughts and Feelings:**

1. Notice any emotional responses or thoughts that arise as you speak. Acknowledge them without judgment.

2. If negative thoughts surface, gently challenge them with compassionate responses.

**Concluding the Session:**

1. End your mirror work with a moment of gratitude towards yourself for taking this time.

2. Take a few deep breaths and gently transition away from the mirror, carrying the sense of self-compassion with you.

## Specific need or Challenge

### Affirmations

- 
- 
- 
- 
- 
- 

- 
- 
- 
- 
- 
- 

## Specific need or Challenge

### Affirmations

- 
- 
- 
- 
- 
- 

- 
- 
- 
- 
- 
- 

## Specific need or Challenge

### Affirmations

- 
- 
- 
- 
- 
- 

- 
- 
- 
- 
- 
-

# ENHANCING EMOTIONAL AWARENESS

## JOURNAL PROMPTS FOR ENHANCING EMOTIONAL AWARENESS

### Physical Sensations of Emotions

"Choose one emotion I felt today and describe where in my body I felt it. What physical sensations accompanied this emotion?"

## JOURNAL PROMPTS FOR ENHANCING EMOTIONAL AWARENESS

### Patterns of Emotional Response

"Looking back over the past month, can I identify any patterns in my emotional responses? What situations, people, or thoughts tend to trigger similar emotions?"

## JOURNAL PROMPTS FOR ENHANCING EMOTIONAL AWARENESS

### Managing Difficult Emotions

"Think of a time recently when I managed a difficult emotion effectively. What strategies did I use, and how did they help?"

# ENHANCING EMOTIONAL AWARENESS

## JOURNAL PROMPTS FOR ENHANCING EMOTIONAL AWARENESS

### Emotions and Decision-Making

"Reflect on a recent decision I made. How did my emotions influence my decision-making process, and would I do anything differently now?"

# BOOSTING MOOD AND ENERGY

## CARDIOVASCULAR EXERCISES

Cardiovascular exercises are a dynamic component of somatic therapy that can significantly enhance mood and energy levels. Activities like light jogging, dancing, or aerobic exercises stimulate the release of endorphins, the body's natural mood elevators. Integrating cardiovascular movements into somatic therapy allows you not only to engage in physical activity but also to become more attuned to the joyful and energizing sensations within your bodies.

### Objectives

To activate the body's natural endorphin release, promoting mood enhancement and a sense of well-being.

To encourage a positive mind-body interaction and awareness that supports emotional health.

### Preparation

Choose a form of cardiovascular exercise that you enjoy and that suits your fitness level, such as brisk walking, light jogging, dancing, or a structured aerobic routine.

Set a goal for the duration and intensity of the exercise that is challenging yet attainable.

### Tips & Advice

Select activities that you find enjoyable, as pleasure in movement is key to sustaining exercise routines and enhancing mood.

Listen to your body, and adjust the intensity and duration of exercises to match your energy levels and mood on any given day.

Remember that consistency is more valuable than intensity.

### Step-by-Step Instructions

1. **Warm-Up:**
   1. Begin with a 5 to 10-minute warm-up to prepare your body for increased activity. This could include gentle stretching or a slower version of your chosen exercise.

**Engage in Cardiovascular Activity:**
   1. Start your chosen exercise at a low to moderate intensity, focusing on the rhythm of your movements and breath.
   2. As you move, pay attention to how your body feels, noticing areas of tension and the sensation of release as you continue.

**Mindful Movement:**
   1. Maintain a mindful presence during the exercise, observing the physical sensations and emotional feelings that arise.
   2. If your mind wanders, gently bring your attention back to your body and the movement, reconnecting with the present moment.

**Cool Down and Reflect:**
   1. Gradually decrease the intensity of your activity, transitioning into a cool-down period with slower movements and deeper breathing.
   2. Reflect on the experience, noting any changes in your mood or energy levels since beginning the exercise.

**Integration:**
   1. Following your cool down, take a few moments to stand or sit quietly, integrating the physical activity with a sense of mental and emotional rejuvenation.
   2. Acknowledge the effort you put into the session and the positive effects it has on your mood and energy.

## LAUGHTER YOGA SESSIONS

Laughter Yoga Sessions offer an unconventional yet highly effective exercise that combines the joyful act of laughing with yogic breathing techniques to promote health, boost mood, and increase energy levels. This unique practice is based on the premise that voluntary laughter provides the same physiological and psychological benefits as spontaneous laughter. Incorporate laughter yoga into your daily routine, even a few minutes a day can have a significant positive impact on your mood and well-being.

### Objectives

To improve overall energy levels and reduce stress through laughter-induced endorphin release.

To encourage social connection and a sense of community by participating in group laughter exercises.

### Preparation

Find a comfortable, private space if practicing alone, or a safe, open area if participating in a group session.

Wear comfortable clothing that doesn't restrict movement or breathing.

Prepare to let go of inhibitions and be open to the experience, regardless of how silly it might feel initially.

### Tips & Advice

Remember, the goal is not humor but the act of laughing itself; allow laughter to flow freely without needing a reason.

Practice regularly to cultivate a habit of laughter in daily life, enhancing resilience to stress.

Explore local or online laughter yoga groups to enjoy the added benefit of social connection.

### Step-by-Step Instructions

**Warm-Up:**

1. Begin with gentle stretching and deep breathing exercises to relax the body and prepare for laughter.

2. Incorporate facial exercises, like smiling broadly and making exaggerated facial expressions, to warm up your laughter muscles.

**Laughter Exercises:**

1. Start with short, forced laughs, gradually allowing them to become longer and more genuine. Use eye contact (if in a group) to encourage contagious laughter.

2. Incorporate playful activities or imaginary scenarios that can induce laughter, such as mimicking funny animal sounds or pretending to laugh while holding different poses.

**Breathing and Relaxation:**

1. Intersperse laughter with deep yogic breathing to maintain balance and ensure oxygenation.

2. Yogic Breathing: Begin with a deep, controlled, and slow inhalation, allowing your abdomen to expand first, followed by your ribcage, and finally filling your upper chest with air. Then, engage in a deep, controlled, and slow exhalation, releasing air starting from your upper chest, moving through your ribcage, and concluding with drawing your abdomen in to fully empty your lungs.

3. After a series of laughter exercises, transition to a relaxation phase. Lie down or sit comfortably, close your eyes, and take deep breaths, allowing the body to relax and absorb the joy and lightness generated by the laughter.

**Closing Reflection:**

1. Conclude the session with a moment of gratitude for the laughter and joy experienced. Reflect on any changes in your mood and energy levels, noting how the act of laughing made you feel.

# PROMOTING RELAXATION AND SLEEP QUALITY

## BREATHWORK EXERCISE FOR CALMING THE NERVOUS SYSTEM

Breathwork is a powerful tool for calming the nervous system and reducing stress. This guided exercise focuses on deep, controlled breathing to activate the parasympathetic nervous system, often referred to as the 'rest and digest' system, promoting relaxation and a sense of calm.

Practice this breathwork exercise daily, or whenever you feel the need to calm your nervous system.

### Objectives

To calm the mind and relax the body.

To activate the parasympathetic nervous system, reducing stress and anxiety.

To improve focus and mental clarity.

### Preparation

Find a quiet, comfortable place where you can sit or lie down without being disturbed.

Wear comfortable clothing that doesn't restrict your breathing.

Decide on a duration for your practice. Even a few minutes can be beneficial.

### Tips & Advice

Be patient with yourself. If you find your mind wandering, gently bring your focus back to your breath.

If you feel dizzy or uncomfortable at any point, return to your normal breathing pattern.

You can vary the length of inhales and exhales as per your comfort, but always ensure a relaxed and full breath.

### Step-by-Step Instructions

**Starting Position:**

1. Sit comfortably with your back straight or lie down on your back. Place one hand on your chest and the other on your abdomen to be more aware of your breathing.

**Focusing on the Breath:**

1. Close your eyes gently. Begin to focus on your natural breathing pattern without trying to change it. Notice the rise and fall of your chest and abdomen.

2. Now, gradually start to deepen your breaths. Inhale slowly through your nose, allowing your abdomen to expand fully, then your chest.

**Controlled Breathing:**

1. Exhale slowly and fully through your mouth. As you exhale, feel your body becoming more relaxed and calm.

2. Try to make your exhale slightly longer than your inhale. For example, if you inhale for a count of four, try to exhale for a count of six.

**Mindful Awareness:**

1. As you continue with this breathing pattern, pay attention to the sensations in your body. Notice the feeling of air entering and leaving your nostrils, the movement of your hands with each breath, and any areas of tension releasing with each exhale.

**Returning to Normal Breathing:**

1. After practicing this breathwork for your chosen duration, gradually let your breathing return to its natural rhythm.

2. Take a moment to sit or lie still, noticing the calmness in your mind and the relaxation in your body.

**Closing the Exercise:**

1. Gently wiggle your fingers and toes, bringing some movement back to your body.

2. Open your eyes slowly and take a moment to transition back to your surroundings.

# Reflection

**Reflect on how you feel after the exercise. Do you notice any changes in your stress levels, thoughts, or physical sensations?**

# Application

**Consider how you might use this breathwork technique in everyday situations when you feel stressed or overwhelmed.**

# ENHANCING RESILIENCE AND SELF-ESTEEM

## POSITIVE AFFIRMATION EXERCISES

Positive Affirmation Exercises blend the physical movement of the body with the transformative power of positive self-talk, a technique that aligns closely with the principles of somatic therapy. This integration facilitates a deeper connection between the mind and the body, reinforcing the somatic experience with empowering cognitions. Engage as often as needed. Daily practice can be especially beneficial for reinforcing positive self-perception and enhancing the somatic healing process.

## Objectives

To reinforce the healing connection between mind and body.

To install a sense of strength and self-compassion during movement.

To address and transform negative somatic experiences into positive bodily awareness.

## Preparation

Select affirmations that resonate with your personal goals and feelings you wish to cultivate, such as "I am strong," "I am at peace," or "I trust in my body's wisdom."

Choose a series of gentle, repetitive movements that you can perform comfortably, such as walking, yoga poses, or stretching exercises.

Create a calm and distraction-free environment.

## Tips & Advice

Choose affirmations that truly resonate with you and reflect your intentions or desired state of being.

Practice regularly to reinforce the positive neural pathways associated with your affirmations.

Be patient and kind to yourself as you integrate this practice into your your somatic therapy healing journey.

## Step-by-Step Instructions

**Establishing Your Movement Pattern:**

1. Begin with simple movements that allow for rhythmic repetition and can be easily synchronized with your breath.

2. The movements should be gentle enough to maintain for the duration of the exercise without causing strain.

**Integrating Affirmations:**

1. As you move, begin to repeat your chosen affirmations aloud or silently. Sync the rhythm of the affirmations with your movement and breath.

2. Focus on the meaning of the words and allow them to resonate with each motion, creating a powerful mind-body connection.

**Maintaining Flow and Focus:**

1. If your mind wanders or doubts emerge, acknowledge them without judgment and gently redirect your attention back to your affirmations and movements.

2. Visualize the positive impact of the affirmations on your body, imagining a warm or healing light accompanying each word and movement.

**Amplifying the Positive Experience:**

1. With each repetition, seek to deepen the emotional resonance of the affirmations, allowing them to become more ingrained in your physical experience.

2. Feel the positive emotions associated with your affirmations and let them permeate your being with each movement.

**Concluding the Exercise:**

1. Gradually wind down your movements, continuing to repeat your affirmations until you come to a natural stop.

## Gentle Exercises

## Affirmations

- 
- 
- 
- 
- 
- 
- 

- 
- 
- 
- 
- 
- 
- 

## Gentle Exercises

## Affirmations

- 
- 
- 
- 
- 
- 
- 

- 
- 
- 
- 
- 
- 
- 

## Gentle Exercises

## Affirmations

- 
- 
- 
- 
- 
- 
- 

- 
- 
- 
- 
- 
- 
-

# ENHANCING RESILIENCE AND SELF-ESTEEM

## SELF-HUG FOR COMFORT AND SAFETY

The Self-Hug for Comfort and Safety is a simple yet profound exercise designed to promote feelings of security, warmth, and self-compassion. This practice leverages the power of physical touch to create a tangible sense of comfort and reassurance, grounding you in moments of distress or disconnection. Integrate the self-hug into your daily routine, or as often as needed, to maintain a sense of inner safety and comfort. It can be particularly beneficial during times of heightened stress or emotional turmoil.

### Objectives

To cultivate a sense of safety and comfort through self-soothing physical touch.

To reinforce feelings of self-love, acceptance, and compassion.

To provide an immediate, accessible tool for emotional regulation and grounding.

### Preparation

Find a quiet, comfortable space where you can be alone and undisturbed.

Stand, sit, or lie down in a position that feels natural and relaxed to you.

Take a few deep breaths to center yourself and become present in the moment.

### Tips & Advice

Practice the self-hug regularly, especially during moments of stress, anxiety, or when you need a reminder of your own support and compassion.

Experiment with variations, such as rubbing your arms for warmth or rocking gently, to find what offers the most comfort.

Remember, the self-hug is a powerful tool for self-care that you can use anytime, anywhere.

### Step-by-Step Instructions

**Initiating the Self-Hug:**

1. Gently wrap your arms around your body, crossing them over your chest. If sitting or lying down, adjust your arms to find the most comforting position.

2. Close your eyes if it feels comfortable, and take a deep, slow breath in and out.

**Deepening the Hug:**

1. Squeeze yourself with as much gentleness or firmness as you need in this moment. Feel the warmth of your own embrace.

2. With each inhale, imagine drawing in warmth, safety, and comfort. With each exhale, release any tension, fear, or sadness you may be holding.

**Adding Affirmations:**

1. Silently or softly say affirmations that reinforce self-compassion and comfort, such as "I am here for myself," "I am worthy of love and care," or "I am safe and supported."

**Maintaining the Embrace:**

1. Stay in this self-hug for as long as you need, continuing to breathe deeply and repeat your affirmations. Notice how your body and emotions respond to the gesture.

**Releasing the Hug:**

1. When you're ready, gently release your arms, letting them fall to your sides. Take a moment to reflect on any changes in your emotional or physical state.

**Immediate Reflection:**

1. Immediately after completing the exercise, take a few moments to sit quietly. Notice any shifts in your emotional state or physical sensations. How do you feel compared to before the exercise?

# ENHANCING RESILIENCE AND SELF-ESTEEM

## POSITIVE MEMORY VISUALIZATION

Positive Memory Visualization is a powerful exercise aimed at enhancing resilience and self-esteem by reconnecting you with moments of strength, joy, and achievement. By vividly recalling positive experiences, you can shift your focus from present challenges to a more empowered and confident state of mind. Incorporate this exercise into your routine as needed, aiming for at least once a week to maintain a positive and empowered mindset.

## Objectives

To reinforce positive self-perception and boost self-esteem through the recall of empowering memories.

To utilize positive memories as a source of resilience in facing current and future challenges.

To strengthen emotional regulation by fostering positive emotional experiences.

## Preparation

Find a quiet, comfortable space where you can relax without distractions.

Have a journal or notepad ready for any insights or feelings you wish to record after the visualization.

Choose a positive memory that evokes feelings of happiness, pride, or accomplishment.

## Tips & Advice

Practice this exercise regularly, especially during times of self-doubt or challenge, to remind yourself of your strengths and achievements.

Try visualizing different positive memories to explore various aspects of your resilience and self-esteem.

## Step-by-Step Instructions

### Relaxation and Centering:

1. Begin by taking several deep, calming breaths. Allow your body to relax with each exhale. Close your eyes gently and continue breathing slowly, preparing your mind for visualization.

### Recalling a Positive Memory:

1. Bring to mind a positive memory that makes you feel happy, proud, or accomplished. This could be a personal achievement, a meaningful connection, or a moment of joy.

2. Visualize this memory as vividly as possible. Imagine the setting, the people involved, the sounds, and the smells. Most importantly, tune into how you felt during this moment.

### Engaging with the Memory:

1. As you immerse yourself in this memory, pay attention to the emotions and physical sensations that arise. Notice the warmth, the energy, or the sense of fulfillment in your body. Reflect on the qualities and strengths you demonstrated in this memory. Acknowledge your capabilities and the positive attributes that led to this moment.

### Drawing Strength from the Memory:

1. Consider how the strengths and emotions from this memory can be applied to your current life situations. How does recalling this moment change your feelings about yourself and your ability to handle challenges?

2. Affirm to yourself that the same qualities that brought you success or joy in the past are still a part of you.

### Reflection and Journaling:

1. Take some time to journal about the memory you chose, the strengths you identified, and how you can apply these insights to enhance your resilience and self-esteem.

# RESILIENCE-BUILDING ACTIVITIES

Building resilience involves developing the capacity to bounce back from adversity, stress, and life's challenges. Resilience is not just about enduring difficulties, but also growing and finding meaning in them. It helps enhance the ability to cope with and recover from difficult experiences and build skills that support adaptability and emotional strength.

Remember that resilience is not about never failing or feeling down; it's about learning and bouncing back.

Be patient and kind to yourself as you work on building resilience. It's a skill that takes time to develop. Don't forget to recognize and celebrate your progress along the way, no matter how small.

### Today's Chosen Goal

### Chosen Activity

### Day or Days of Practice

### Chosen Time

### Chosen Space

## JOURNALING ON PAST CHALLENGES

1. Reflect on a past challenge and write about how you coped with it. Focus on what you learned from the experience and how it has contributed to your growth.

2. Identify the strengths and skills that helped you overcome that challenge. Consider how you can apply these strengths to current or future difficulties.

## GOAL SETTING

1. Set a realistic, achievable goal for yourself. This could be related to personal development, a hobby, or a professional aspiration.

2. Break down the goal into small, manageable steps and track your progress. Celebrate small victories along the way.

3. Reflect on the journey towards your goal, noting how overcoming obstacles and setbacks contributes to your resilience.

## MINDFULNESS AND GRATITUDE

1. Engage in daily mindfulness practices, such as meditation or mindful walking, to enhance present-moment awareness and reduce stress.

2. Keep a gratitude journal, noting three things you are grateful for each day. This practice helps shift focus from problems to positives.

## BUILDING A SUPPORT NETWORK

1. Actively work on building or strengthening your support network. Connect with friends, family, or groups who provide emotional support.

2. Practice being open and vulnerable with trusted individuals. Sharing your challenges and receiving support can significantly bolster resilience.

## PROBLEM-SOLVING SKILLS

1. When faced with a problem, practice approaching it with a problem-solving mindset: Break the problem down, brainstorm potential solutions, and evaluate their feasibility.

2. Taking proactive steps, even small ones, in solving problems can reinforce a sense of control and resilience.

## SELF-TALK

1. Cultivate a habit of positive self-talk. Challenge negative or pessimistic thoughts by reframing them into more positive and realistic ones.

2. Use affirmations to reinforce resilience, such as "I am capable of handling life's challenges" or "I grow stronger with each obstacle I overcome."

# SELF-COMPASSION PRACTICES

Self-compassion involves treating yourself with the same kindness, concern, and support you'd offer to a good friend. Cultivating self-compassion can lead to increased resilience, reduced anxiety and depression, and more positive overall well-being.

Remember that being compassionate towards yourself doesn't mean you are being self-indulgent or selfish.

Engage in these self-compassion practices daily. Consistency is key to rewiring habitual patterns of self-criticism. Self-compassion is a skill that develops over time.

Choose a time when you are unlikely to be disturbed, allowing for focus and introspection. And, have a journal or notebook handy for any reflective writing you might wish to do.

Be patient with yourself. Cultivating self-compassion can be challenging, especially if you are used to self-criticism.

### Chosen Activity

### Day or Days of Practice

### Chosen Time

### Chosen Space

## MINDFUL SELF-COMPASSION BREAK

1. Whenever you notice you are experiencing stress or emotional discomfort, pause and acknowledge that this is a difficult moment.

2. Place your hand over your heart or another soothing place and say to yourself, "This is hard right now. How can I care for and comfort myself in this moment?"

3. Use kind and understanding language towards yourself, acknowledging that suffering is a part of the human experience.

## SELF-COMPASSION JOURNALING

1. Spend a few minutes each day writing down things you did well, however small. Acknowledge your efforts rather than focusing solely on outcomes.

2. Write down kind words to yourself, especially in areas where you feel lacking. Treat yourself as you would a dear friend.

## LOVING-KINDNESS MEDITATION

**28-DAY SOMATIC PLAN DAY 16**

1. Begin by finding a comfortable position and closing your eyes. Focus on your breath for a few moments.

2. Silently repeat phrases of loving-kindness towards yourself, such as "May I be happy. May I be healthy. May I be safe. May I live with ease."

3. Gradually extend these wishes to others, starting from loved ones to neutral individuals, and eventually to all beings.

## SELF-COMPASSION AFFIRMATIONS

1. Create affirmations that reinforce self-compassion. For example, "I am worthy of kindness," or "I accept myself as I am."

2. Repeat these affirmations daily, especially during times of self-criticism or challenge.

## GRATITUDE REFLECTIONS

1. Regularly reflect on aspects of yourself and your life that you are grateful for.

2. Recognize your strengths, achievements, and the support you receive from others.

# NURTURING MIND-BODY CONNECTION

## MINDFULNESS EXERCISES FOR EVERYDAY LIFE

Mindfulness is the practice of being fully present and engaged in the moment, aware of your thoughts and feelings without distraction or judgment. Incorporating mindfulness into everyday life can enhance emotional regulation, reduce stress, and improve overall well-being.

Aim to engage in this mindfulness exercise daily. Over time, try to expand mindfulness to more activities and longer durations.

## Objectives

To cultivate a regular practice of mindfulness in daily activities.

To develop greater awareness of the present moment, reducing habitual patterns of stress and reactivity.

To enhance concentration, patience, and a sense of calm in everyday life.

## Preparation

Choose an activity you perform daily as the focus for your mindfulness practice. This could be something as simple as brushing your teeth, eating a meal, walking, or doing household chores.

Approach the activity with the intention of being fully present and attentive.

## Tips & Advice

Start with short, simple activities and gradually incorporate mindfulness into more aspects of your day.

Practice regularly. The more you practice mindfulness, the more natural it will become.

Be patient and kind to yourself. Mindfulness is a skill that takes time to develop.

## Step by Step Instructions

**Mindful Breathing:**

1. Begin by taking a few deep breaths, focusing your attention solely on the sensation of breathing.

2. Notice the air entering and leaving your nostrils, the rise and fall of your chest, and the rhythm of your breath.

**Engaging in the Chosen Activity:**

1. As you start your chosen activity, aim to be fully present with it. For example, if you are eating, focus on the taste, texture, and aroma of the food.

2. If your mind wanders, gently bring your attention back to the activity.

**Observing Thoughts and Sensations:**

1. Observe any thoughts or feelings that arise without judgment. Acknowledge them and then return your focus to the present moment.

2. Pay attention to the physical sensations associated with the activity. Notice the movements of your body, the contact with objects, and any sensory experiences.

**Reflecting on the Experience:**

1. After completing the activity, take a moment to reflect on the experience. Did you notice anything new or different by being fully present?

2. Consider how this mindful approach made you feel. Did you find it calming, challenging, or enlightening?

# TECHNIQUES FOR CULTIVATING PRESENT-MOMENT AWARENESS

Cultivating present-moment awareness is a fundamental aspect of mindfulness and meditation practices.

This kind of awareness helps you stay grounded in the current moment, reducing stress and increasing contentment. Cultivating present-moment awareness is a skill that requires regular practice. By incorporating these techniques into your daily life, you can enhance your ability to live more mindfully and enjoy the richness of the present moment.

Here are several techniques that can be employed to cultivate present-moment awareness:

## MINDFUL BREATHING

1. Focus on your breath, noticing the sensation of air entering and leaving your nostrils, or the rise and fall of your chest or abdomen.
2. When your mind wanders, gently bring your attention back to your breath.

## BODY SCAN MEDITATION

*28-DAY SOMATIC PLAN DAY 1*

1. Slowly direct your attention through different parts of your body, starting from the toes and moving upwards.
2. Notice any sensations, tension, or discomfort without judgment, simply observing and acknowledging.

## MINDFUL OBSERVATION

1. Choose an object within your environment and focus all your attention on it.
2. Notice its shape, color, texture, and any other qualities without attaching labels or judgments.

## MINDFUL LISTENING

1. Pay attention to the sounds in your environment, whether it's birds chirping, the hum of a refrigerator, or distant traffic.
2. Listen without labeling or identifying the sources of the sounds.

## MINDFUL EATING

1. Eat slowly and intentionally, paying attention to the taste, texture, and smell of your food.
2. Notice the physical sensations of eating and your body's response.

## WALKING MEDITATION

*28-DAY SOMATIC PLAN DAY 5*

1. Walk slowly, and focus on the sensation of your feet touching the ground.
2. Be aware of your body's movements and how it feels to move through space.

## MINDFUL DAILY ACTIVITIES

1. Engage fully with routine activities, like brushing your teeth or washing dishes.
2. Pay attention to every detail of the activity instead of doing it on autopilot.

## GRATITUDE PRACTICE

1. Regularly reflect on things you're grateful for.
2. This can shift your focus to the present and what you appreciate in your current life.

## USE OF REMINDERS

1. Set periodic reminders throughout the day to pause and bring your focus back to the present.
2. This could be through an app, a note, or even a specific chime.

## GUIDED IMAGERY

1. Use visualization techniques to imagine a peaceful and calming scene.
2. This helps in anchoring your mind in the present and letting go of worries about the past or future.

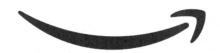

# Healing Together

As you work through these pages, I hope you're finding moments of insight, empowerment, and self-discovery that resonate deeply with you.

I know you're busy, and I truly appreciate your time.

If you could spare just two minutes to share your thoughts with a review on Amazon, it would mean a great deal to me.

Just scan the QR code above, and you'll land directly on the book review page. It's that easy!

Your feedback could help me make the book even better, and might even encourage someone else to pick it up. Who knows? It might change their life just like it might have changed yours.

Thank you for considering this small but significant way of giving back.

I appreciate it immensely.

Ashley

# ENHANCE YOUR SOMATIC WORKOUT EXPERIENCE BY EMBRACING THE OUTDOORS

I recommend finding a quiet spot, perhaps under a shady tree or in a small park, to engage with your exercises while breathing in fresh air.

*Why?*

Taking your somatic workout outdoors can really transform your experience!

Imagine doing your exercises surrounded by nature.

Not only does it help you connect deeply with the environment, but it also works wonders in melting away stress and boosting your mood. There's something about fresh air that makes breathing exercises feel even more revitalizing. Plus, being outside gives you a healthy dose of Vitamin D from natural sunlight – great for your overall health.

Scan the QR code to download and print your A4 workout sheets and get access to the videos. These sheets are not only more practical than a traditional book format, but their portability also allows you to easily move and bring them closer during your exercises.

With the convenience of these easy-to-handle sheets, you can effortlessly track your progress, jot down reflections, and fully immerse yourself in your practice, wherever you choose to be.

### PROMOTING RELAXATION & SLEEP QUALITY

**Restorative Yoga Poses**

Legs Up The Wall

Corpse Pose

Bound Angle Pose

Spinal Twist

**Gentle Stretching**

### ENHANCING EMOTIONAL AWARNESS

**Somatic Dancing**

**Vibrational Movement**

### NURTURING MIND-BODY CONNECTION

**Somatic Pilates**

**Tai Chi or Qigong**

**Feldenkrais Method**

# ENHANCE YOUR SOMATIC WORKOUT EXPERIENCE BY EMBRACING THE OUTDOORS

## HOLISTIC TENSION RELEASE

**Somatic Yoga Poses**
Warrior III
Eagle Pose
Tree Pose

**Gentle Somatic Yoga Poses**
Cat and Caw
Child Pose
Supine Twist
Seated Forward Bend

**Balancing Exercises**

**Tai Chi Movements**

**Psoas Release Exercises**

## ENHANCING RESILIENCE & SELF-ESTEEM

**Empowerment Yoga Poses**
Mountain Pose with Arm Raises
Worrior I

**Pelvic Tilts**

**Hip Circles**

## MANAGING SYMPTOMS OF ANXIETY

**Walking Meditation**

**Qigong Exercises**

## BOOSTING MOOD & ENERGY

**Power Yoga Poses**
Warrior II
Cobra Pose
Chair Pose
Plank Pose
Somatic Bridge Pose

**Dynamic Stretching**

## WORKING THROUGH TRAUMA

**Yoga Poses for Grief**
Constructive Rest Position
Butterfly Pose Forward fall
Seated Forward Bend
Wind Relieving Pose

## DOWNLOAD THE BONUS MATERIAL (PAGE 5)

The meditation and the hypnotherapy track will deepen your experience and enhance the effectiveness of the entire program.

**Warning needed to not use the hypnotherapy track while driving or operating machinery.**

# HOW IT WORKS

This program is designed to offer a holistic approach to somatic therapy, blending physical exercises with mental and emotional reflective activities. The aim is to foster greater self-awareness, emotional resilience, and physical well-being throughout this guided 28-day journey. As each week unfolds, you'll encounter new layers of self-discovery, starting from foundational awareness, moving through exploration and movement, advancing towards emotional processing, and finally culminating in integration and growth. Before you begin, I recommend taking a sneak peek at the exercises and activities planned for each day. This preparatory step will help you mentally prepare for what's ahead, smoothing out any potential bumps by giving you a clear idea of each exercise.

I suggest keeping your journal close at hand. Before starting each day's activity, take a moment to jot down your current feelings and thoughts. After the activity, reflect on any changes or insights; ask yourself, "What shifted within me?". Pay attention to subtle changes in your body, thoughts, or emotions. This brief check-in will deepen your journey, helping you identify patterns, shifts, and progress. For this you can refer to the Progress Tracking Chart at page 46. Embrace flexibility in your approach, remain open to the experiences as they come, and remember, this journey is yours to shape. Feel free to adjust the intensity and duration of each activity to your comfort level.

Here's how to prepare for the program with additional activities:

- Consider what you wish to achieve through this journey and record these goals in a journal.
- Identify a comfortable spot where you can relax and move around easily. This will become your sanctuary for the sessions.
- Ensure you have a yoga mat, comfortable clothes, and a journal handy. You'll want to be comfortable and ready to capture your thoughts.
- Choose a specific time each day for your sessions. Consistency is crucial.
- Incorporate small mindfulness exercises into your daily routine, such as focusing on your breath for a few minutes.
- Write down some positive affirmations to motivate you throughout the days ahead.
- Familiarize yourself with the basics of somatic therapy to better understand what you're diving into.

Each step, each breath, and each moment of reflection is an opportunity to connect more deeply with yourself, discover strength, resilience, and a deeper sense of peace.

| 1 | BODY SCAN MEDITATION (10 MIN) + JOURNALING REFLECTION (5 MIN) | WORKBOOK, p. 99 |
|---|---|---|
| 2 | GENTLE SOMATIC YOGA (15 MIN) | SOMATIC SHEETS p.34 |
| 3 | EXERCISE TO CONNECT WITH THE PRESENT (5 MIN) + BODY INTUITION (10 MIN) | WORKBOOK p. 42 & 44 |
| 4 | PHYSICAL GROUNDING EXERCISE (5 MIN) + BOUND ANGLE POSE (10 MIN) | WORKBOOK, p. 77 SOMATIC SHEETS p.12 |
| 5 | WALKING MEDITATION (15 MIN) | SOMATIC SHEETS p.54 OR WORKBOOK, p. 99 |
| 6 | BREATHING EXERCISE FOR PAIN RELIEF + DYNAMIC TENSION AND RELEASE | WORKBOOK, p.68 & 66 |
| 7 | EXERCISE FOR RELEASING TRAUMATIC ENERGY STORED IN THE BODY (15 MIN) | WORKBOOK, p.52 |
| 8 | GROUNDING WITH THE 5 SENSES (5 MIN) + VOCAL TONING AND HUMMING (10 MIN) | WORKBOOK, p.77 & 70 |
| 9 | IDENTIFY AND EXPRESSING EMOTIONS THROUGH THE BODY (15 MIN) | WORKBOOK, p.54 |
| 10 | SHAKING/VIBRATIONAL MOVEMENT (15 MIN) - Use the Ecstatic Dance music BONUS | SOMATIC SHEETS p.80 |
| 11 | GENTLE SOMATIC YOGA (15 MIN) | SOMATIC SHEETS p.34 |
| 12 | QIGONG PRACTICE (15 MIN) | SOMATIC SHEETS p.56 |
| 13 | SOMATIC DANCING (15 MIN) - Use the Ecstatic Dance music BONUS | SOMATIC SHEETS p.78 |
| 14 | YOGA POSES FOR GRIEF (15 MIN) | SOMATIC SHEETS p.1 |
| 15 | SHAKING/VIBRATIONAL MOVEMENT (15 MIN) - Use the Ecstatic Dance music BONUS | SOMATIC SHEETS p.80 |
| 16 | CONCENTRATION MEDITATION (10 MNS) | WORKBOOK p. 72 |
| 17 | PSOAS RELEASE EXERCISES (15 MIN) | SOMATIC SHEETS p.44 |
| 18 | SOMATIC BREATHING (10 MIN) + MINDFUL OBSERVATION (5 MIN) | SOMATIC SHEETS p.11 |
| 19 | GENTLE SOMATIC YOGA (15 MIN) | SOMATIC SHEETS p.34 |
| 20 | LAUGHTER YOGA EXERCISE (5 MIN) + JOURNALING AND REFLECTIONS (10 MNS) | WORKBOOK, p.89 |
| 21 | BODY SCAN MEDITATION (10 MIN) + JOURNALING AND REFLECTION (5 MIN) | WORKBOOK, p.80 |
| 22 | SOMATIC PILATES (15 MIN) | SOMATIC SHEETS p.50 |
| 23 | DEEP BREATHING (5 MIN) + POSITIVE AFFIRMATION EXERCISE (10 MIN) | WORKBOOK p.92 |
| 24 | EMPOWERMENT YOGA POSES (10 MIN) + EMPOWERMENT EXERCISES (5 MIN) | SOMATIC SHEETS p.70 |
| 25 | EMOTIONAL AWARENESS JOURNALING (15 MIN) | WORKBOOK, p.40 |
| 26 | FELDENKRAIS METHOD EXERCISES (15 MIN) | SOMATIC SHEETS p.49 |
| 27 | SOMATIC DANCING (15 MIN) | SOMATIC SHEETS p.78 |
| 28 | GENTLE STRETCHING (10 MIN) + MINDFUL BREATHING (5 MIN) | SOMATIC SHEETS p.28 |

# CONCLUSION

As we turn the last page, let's take a moment to honor the journey you're embarking on—a journey toward holistic well-being that holds body awareness at its heart and is cradled within a supportive therapeutic space. By learning to listen—to truly listen—to the wisdom of your body, you begin to unlock the secrets of your inner world. This is where the transformation begins, and this is where you start to weave the narrative of your own resilience.

Picture yourself as both the navigator and the vessel on this voyage. With every breath and beat of your heart, you chart a course through the waters of self-awareness. Your therapist is your lighthouse, casting a steady, understanding light that helps you steer by the stars of empathy and validation.

It's within this sanctuary that you'll find the courage to delve into the tapestry of your emotions and experiences, guided by somatic practices that help to process, integrate, and ultimately transform. The threads of trauma-informed care weave through this tapestry, ensuring that every pattern—no matter how tangled—can be traced and understood with compassion.

Building resilience is like cultivating a garden within you, where each somatic technique plants a seed of strength and every session under the nurturing presence of your therapist helps it to grow. This garden is where you'll learn to thrive, not just survive, amid life's storms and seasons.

And so, with a spirit of openness and the empowering tools of somatic therapy, you step forward. You are ready to embrace a life enriched by profound self-awareness and emotional resilience—a life where each step is taken with intention, each breath brings you closer to balance, and every day holds the promise of renewed vitality and peace.

This is not just an end; it's a beautiful beginning. It's your journey toward wholeness, and it starts now.

# MORE HEALING BOOKS FROM US...

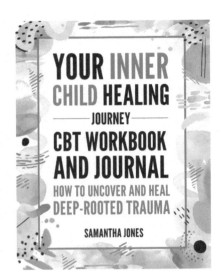

### Your Inner Child Healing Journey

How to Uncover and Heal Deep-Rooted Trauma. A CBT Workbook and Journal to Face Abandonament, Neglet and Abuse, Improve Self-Esteem & Regain Emotional Freedom

Samantha Jones

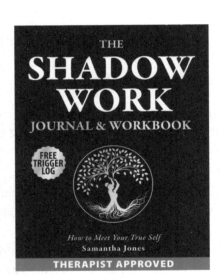

### The Shadow Work Journal & Workbook

How to Meet Your True Self: Integrate & Transcend Your Dark Side through Self-Discovery Exercises. Deep Guided Prompts for Inner Child Soothing, Healing & Growth

Samantha Jones

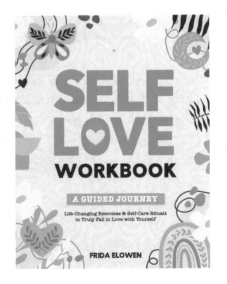

### Self Love Workbook

A Guided Journey with Life-Changing Activities & Self-Care Rituals to Truly Fall in Love with Yourself. Heal Emotional Wounds, Recognize Your Worth & Embrace Your Uniqueness

Frida Elowen

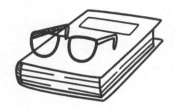

# SOMATIC THERAPY
# RECOMMENDED READING LIST

**The Body Keeps the Score: Brain, Mind, and Body in the Healing of Trauma** by Bessel van der Kolk
A groundbreaking work on understanding and treating traumatic stress.

**Waking the Tiger: Healing Trauma** by Peter A. Levine
Introduces the concept of 'body memory', explaining how the body can heal from trauma through somatic therapy.

**Body Awareness as Healing Therapy: The Case of Nora** by Moshe Feldenkrais
Explores the relationship between movement and consciousness and offers exercises for improved physical and mental health.

**Somatics: Reawakening The Mind's Control Of Movement, Flexibility, And Health** by Thomas Hanna
Details the practice and philosophy of somatics, providing a pathway to reclaim control of one's bodily movements and freedom.

**Embodied Healing: Using Yoga to Recover from Trauma and Extreme Stress** by Lisa Danylchuk
Connects the principles of yoga with somatic therapy for a holistic approach to healing.

**The Body in Psychotherapy: Inquiries in Somatic Psychology** by Don Hanlon Johnson
Delves into the role of the body in psychological care and the significance of body experience in the therapeutic process.

**Trauma and Memory: Brain and Body in a Search for the Living Past** by Peter A. Levine
A closer look at how the body stores memories and how somatic therapy can access and heal these memories.

**Sensing, Feeling, and Action** by Bonnie Bainbridge Cohen
Discusses the development of bodily-kinesthetic intelligence and how awareness of the body can enhance movement and emotion.

**Healing Trauma: A Pioneering Program for Restoring the Wisdom of Your Body** by Peter A. Levine
Offers a step-by-step approach to using somatic experiencing for personal trauma recovery.

**In an Unspoken Voice: How the Body Releases Trauma and Restores Goodness** by Peter A. Levine
Explores the interconnection between psychological and physiological healing processes.